Feminist Reflections on Growth and Transformation: Asian American Women in Therapy

Feminist Reflections on Growth and Transformation: Asian American Women in Therapy has been co-published simultaneously as *Women & Therapy*, Volume 30, Numbers 3/4 2007.

Feminist Reflections on Growth and Transformation: Asian American Women in Therapy

Debra M. Kawahara, PhD
Oliva M. Espín, PhD
Editors

Feminist Reflections on Growth and Transformation: Asian American Women in Therapy has been co-published simultaneously as *Women & Therapy*, Volume 30, Numbers 3/4 2007.

Routledge
Taylor & Francis Group
New York London

Feminist Reflections on Growth and Transformation: Asian American Women in Therapy has been co-published simultaneously as *Women & Therapy*®, Volume 30, Numbers 3/4 2007.

The development, preparation, and publication of this work has been undertaken with great care. However, the publisher, employees, editors, and agents of The Haworth Press and all imprints of The Haworth Press, Inc., including The Haworth Medical Press® and Pharmaceutical Products Press®, are not responsible for any errors contained herein or for consequences that may ensue from use of materials or information contained in this work. With regard to case studies, identities and circumstances of individuals discussed herein have been changed to protect confidentiality. Any resemblance to actual persons, living or dead, is entirely coincidental.

The Haworth Press is committed to the dissemination of ideas and information according to the highest standards of intellectual freedom and the free exchange of ideas. Statements made and opinions expressed in this publication do not necessarily reflect the views of the Publisher, Directors, management, or staff of The Haworth Press, Inc., or an endorsement by them.

First published by

The Haworth Press, Inc., 10 Alice Street, Binghamton, NY 13904-1580 USA

This edition published 2012 by Routledge

Routledge
Taylor & Francis Group
711 Third Avenue
New York, NY 10017

Routledge
Taylor & Francis Group
2 Park Square, Milton Park
Abingdon, Oxon OX14 4RN

Library of Congress Cataloging-in-Publication Data

Kawahara, Debra M.
Feminist reflections on growth and transformation: Asian American women in therapy / Debra M. Kawahara, Oliva M. Espín.
p. cm.
"Co-published simultaneously as Women & Therapy, volume 30, numbers 3/4"
Includes bibliographical references and index.
ISBN-13: 978-0-7890-3433-5 (hard cover: alk. paper)
ISBN-10: 0-7890-3433-6 (hard cover: alk. paper)
ISBN-13: 978-0-7890-3434-2 (soft cover: alk. paper)
ISBN-10: 0-7890-3434-4 (soft cover: alk. paper)
1. Asian American women-Mental health. 2. Feminist therapy. 3. Psychiatry, Transcultural. I. Espín, Oliva M. II. Title. III. Series: Women & therapy.
RC451. 5. A75K39 2007
616. 89' 14082—dc22

2006027882

Feminist Reflections on Growth and Transformation: Asian American Women in Therapy

Debra M. Kawahara, PhD
Oliva M. Espín, PhD
Editors

Feminist Reflections on Growth and Transformation: Asian American Women in Therapy has been co-published simultaneously as *Women & Therapy*, Volume 30, Numbers 3/4 2007.

Routledge
Taylor & Francis Group
New York London

Feminist Reflections on Growth and Transformation: Asian American Women in Therapy has been co-published simultaneously as *Women & Therapy*®, Volume 30, Numbers 3/4 2007.

First published by

The Haworth Press, Inc., 10 Alice Street, Binghamton, NY 13904-1580 USA

This edition published 2012 by Routledge

Routledge
Taylor & Francis Group
711 Third Avenue
New York, NY 10017

Routledge
Taylor & Francis Group
2 Park Square, Milton Park
Abingdon, Oxon OX14 4RN

Library of Congress Cataloging-in-Publication Data

Kawahara, Debra M.
Feminist reflections on growth and transformation: Asian American women in therapy / Debra M. Kawahara, Oliva M. Espín.
p. cm.
"Co-published simultaneously as Women & Therapy, volume 30, numbers 3/4"
Includes bibliographical references and index.
ISBN-13: 978-0-7890-3433-5 (hard cover: alk. paper)
ISBN-10: 0-7890-3433-6 (hard cover: alk. paper)
ISBN-13: 978-0-7890-3434-2 (soft cover: alk. paper)
ISBN-10: 0-7890-3434-4 (soft cover: alk. paper)
1. Asian American women-Mental health. 2. Feminist therapy. 3. Psychiatry, Transcultural. I. Espín, Oliva M. II. Title. III. Series: Women & therapy.
RC451. 5. A75K39 2007
616. 89' 14082—dc22

2006027882

Feminist Reflections on Growth and Transformation: Asian American Women in Therapy

CONTENTS

ABOUT THE EDITORS

Debra M. Kawahara, PhD, is Assistant Professor of Psychology at the California School of Professional Psychology at Alliant International University in San Diego. Her research and professional interests include multicultural and feminist psychology, Asian American mental health, women and leadership, and multicultural competencies in clinical/counseling practice. Dr. Kawahara has numerous publications, focusing on the integration of multicultural and feminist principles in psychotherapy. She has also been an active member and officer for several professional organizations, including the American Psychological Association (APA) and the Asian American Psychological Association (AAPA).

Oliva M. Espín, PhD, is Professor Emerita of Women's Studies at San Diego State University and Psychology at the California School of Professional Psychology at Alliant International University. In her longstanding work as a psychotherapist, teacher, and consultant, Dr. Espín has emphasized work with women. She was a pioneer in the practice and theory of feminist therapy with women from different cultural backgrounds, particularly US-born Latinas and immigrant/refugee women. She has done extensive research, teaching, and training on diversity issues in psychology. She has also served in several boards and committees of the American Psychological Association and other professional organizations.

INTRODUCTION

Asian American Women in Therapy: Feminist Reflections on Growth and Transformations

Debra M. Kawahara
Oliva M. Espín

SUMMARY. The introduction to this special collection provides the framework that underlies all of the articles presented. The complexity and multidimensionality of identity is discussed as well as its relevance to this volume. The group identity of being a woman of Asian ancestry in the U.S. is the common experience that ties all of the articles together. A summary of each of the articles is provided. doi:10.1300/J015v30n03_01

Debra M. Kawahara, PhD, is Assistant Professor in Clinical Psychology, California School of Professional Psychology at Alliant International University and maintains a private practice in San Diego, CA. Oliva M. Espín, PhD, is Professor Emerita in Women's Studies, San Diego State University and Psychology, California School of Professional Psychology at Alliant International University.

Address correspondence to: Debra M. Kawahara, California School of Professional Psychology, Alliant International University, 10455 Pomerado Road, San Diego, CA 92131-1799 USA (E-mail: dkawahara@alliant.edu).

[Haworth co-indexing entry note]: "Asian American Women in Therapy: Feminist Reflections on Growth and Transformations." Kawahara, Debra M., and Oliva M. Espín. Co-published simultaneously in *Women & Therapy* (The Haworth Press, Inc.) Vol. 30, No. 3/4, 2007, pp. 1-5; and: *Feminist Reflections on Growth and Transformation: Asian American Women in Therapy* (ed: Debra M. Kawahara, and Oliva M. Espín) The Haworth Press, Inc., 2007, pp. 1-5. Single or multiple copies of this article are available for a fee from The Haworth Document Delivery Service [1-800-HAWORTH, 9:00 a.m. - 5:00 p.m. (EST). E-mail address: docdelivery@haworthpress.com].

Available online at http://wt.haworthpress.com

doi:10.1300/J015v30n03_01

[Article copies available for a fee from The Haworth Document Delivery Service: 1-800-HAWORTH. E-mail address: <docdelivery@haworthpress.com> Website: <http://www.HaworthPress.com>

KEYWORDS. Asian American, women of color, multicultural counseling, feminist therapy, treatment

As I began this journey, I (Debra) asked myself whether the focus of this special volume on Asian American women and multicultural feminist therapy was still relevant and useful or was it behind the times. When the focus of theories seems to be shifting to intersecting identities and notions of multiple realities, was I hanging onto an archaic framework of understanding race, ethnicity, and gender as salient threads in the interweaving of identity with the other threads of class, religion/spirituality, national origin, immigration status, sexual orientation, and language, to name a few?

Then, the image of a cup of tea emerged for me. Tea has a history dating back to around 2700 B.C. and was thought to have been discovered in China's Sichuan and Yunnan provinces. From the fifth century A.D., its social prominence grew from exportation throughout Asia and Europe. Over the course of time, tea and its rituals have dynamically transformed in relation to the social, political, and cultural context where it was the beverage of choice (Plutschow, 1999). Although tea has general categories such as flavor, clarity, color, and aroma, the diversity among tea variations is influenced by the environmental conditions in which the tea is grown, the age and number of leaves in one's cup, and the final appearance of the tea leaves. In the end, each tea has its own uniqueness and richness and can be distinguished by our five senses of smell, sight, taste, touch, and sound.

Tea can be seen as a multidimensional symbol paralleling identity. Identity also has general categories or social locations in its overall composition such as worldview, beliefs, values, race, ethnicity, gender, sexual orientation, class, age, and religious/spiritual orientation. Like tea, our identity is composed of variations in these social locations based on the contexts and cultures that we have interfaced with, our life experiences and circumstances, and the salience of these multiple dimensions over our lifespan. And similar to tea, part of what makes each of us unique is the specific constellation of these social locations and the interactions between them. For example, my personal experience as an Asian American woman born in the U.S. is different from those in other generational cohorts and different from those experiences of Asian women who are immigrants, lesbians, or mothers. At the same time, I share some similar experiences with these women that I do not share with women who are not of Asian ancestry.

I (Oliva), although not of Asian ancestry and by no means an expert in these populations, felt compelled to become involved in this project by my own desire to learn more and by Debra's passionate interest in relevant issues about psychotherapy with women of Asian backgrounds. Early in my career, concurrent with my growing awareness of the psychological impact of race, culture, and ethnicity, I encountered the feminist movement and found its basic tenets consonant with my own life experience. My long-term interest in the intersections of gender and race brought me to therapy practice and to writing and research with and for women from different ethnic backgrounds. The fact is that we all live as embodied sexualized and racialized beings. At the simplest level, no one can be solely a man or a woman, *except* as a member of some racial group or groups. No one can be a member of a racial or cultural group, *except* as a man or a woman. Femaleness and maleness are unintelligible in isolation from a given race, ethnicity, religious perspective, and other sociocultural contexts. The boundaries of sex are also boundaries of race and vice-versa. These distinct categories are always lived as interconnected by any given individual. Perhaps there are more than two genders. And, as we know, racial categories may be predicated falsely on dichotomies claimed to be biological. Yet–even though these racial and gender dichotomies are more social categories than specific ontological realities–their profound societal and personal consequences form the context of everyday life processes of oppression and privilege, and the lens through which we learn to make human bodies intelligible.

We all have intersecting identities. Within those identities, there are some common beliefs, values, and experiences because of one or more group membership identities. Certainly, this book is based on some common identities that underlie all of the articles. The common group identity of being a woman of Asian descent in the U.S. frames this volume. The power of this group identity is illustrated by the works collected here and is combined with the intersection of other identity dimensions such as ethnicity, immigration status, religion, sexual orientation, and relational status. The focus on women who are members of the Asian race in the U.S. is the common thread throughout all the articles. These articles share perspectives on Asian American women's lived experiences and psychological issues relevant to them as women and as Asian persons. Yet, as always, a caution about overgeneralizing must be made. Hopefully, these articles together will help readers become cognizant of the unique experiences–differences as well as similarities–among Asian and Asian American women due to the constellation of factors that comprise their overall identity.

The overall goal for this collection is to be informative for clinicians: Asian American feminist clinicians, White clinicians, and other interested clinicians who work with these women as well. We intend it to be a contribution to the ongoing process of development of new paradigms for understanding human variability and diversity in ways of knowing and living.

In the first section, the articles by Jean Lau Chin and Debra Kawahara illustrate Asian American women who are powerful and strong, countering the historically long-standing stereotypes of Asian American women as passive, docile, and subservient. The Asian American women in both of these articles are portrayed as empowered agents in their own personal and professional worlds.

The next set of articles focuses on the construction of identity. Sung Ha Suh discusses the considerations and conflicts that Asian American women face when defining their gender identity. Neesha Patel examines the social construction of South Asian womanhood in the context of the U.S. and South Asian communities, while Patricia Heras discusses cultural and identity issues relevant for therapy with second generation Filipinas. Irene Chung illustrates emotional parity negotiations in marital relationships for Chinese immigrant women using examples of clients from her own private practice.

Further clinical issues are addressed by Eliza Noh who paradoxically reframes the act of suicide as a means of agency rather than just a cry for help, while highlighting the inherent problems in societal systems that contribute to the women's emotional states. Diya Kallivayalil examines South Asian immigrant women survivors of domestic violence and provides illustrations of South Asian practitioners' effective use of feminist and multicultural principles. Next, Suzanne Dibble, Noriko Sato, and Ellen Haller present results from a pilot study on Asian American lesbians, dispelling beliefs of poor physical health among lesbians and highlighting some interesting mental health implications from their results. The article by Julia Ting and Wei-Chin Hwang presents a conceptual framework that integrates multiculturalism and feminism in understanding and treating eating disorders among Asian American women.

The next section focuses on specific therapeutic approaches that can be considered when working with Asian American women. Neha Navsaria and Suni Petersen provide an innovative therapeutic approach based on Hindu understandings of Shakti. Their experiences using this as an effective tool in therapy with immigrant and second-generation Hindu Indian women are highlighted. Kayoko Yokoyama presents a variety of multiculturally informed feminist therapeutic approaches to work on body image and eating disorders among Asian American women. Yuli Liu, Yuying Tsong, and Diane Hayashino discuss a framework for group counseling with Asian American women that incorporates multiculturalism and feminism as well as discuss their experiences as facilitators of such groups.

Finally, this special collection would not be complete without addressing the training of multicultural feminist therapy practitioners to work with these populations. Karen Suyemoto and Joan Liem with contributions from Jennifer Kuhn, Elizabeth Mongillo, and Jesse Tauriac focus on training therapists to develop cultural competence. Three key training experiences–developing cultural self-awareness, acquiring knowledge, and refining clinical skills using a reflexive approach–are presented by these authors. Narratives from trainees' experiences illustrate the impact of these experiences on their professional and personal development.

As we began this volume, we intentionally wanted a diversity of identities, experiences, and histories, especially those of women from Asian populations who have not been well-represented in the literature. We hope that this collection of articles contributes to increasing the knowledge and skills that will assist clinicians in working more effectively with female clients of Asian ancestry. Our wish is that the experiences of those whose voices remain less heard will continue to be explored in the future.

We now invite you to sit back and enjoy these works with a hot cup of tea.

REFERENCE

Plutschow, H. (1999). An anthropological perspective on the Japanese tea ceremony. *Anthropoetics*, *5*. Retrieved July 2, 2005, from http://www.humnet.ucla.edu/humnet/anthropoetics/ap0501/tea.htm

doi:10.1300/J015v30n03_01

ASIAN AMERICAN WOMEN'S PORTRAITS OF EMPOWERMENT

Psychotherapy for Asian American Woman Warriors

Jean Lau Chin

SUMMARY. To treat Asian American women in psychotherapy, one needs to be cognizant of the images they conjure up. Negative images common in the media and literature need to be replaced by empowering ones if we are to be responsive to multicultural and feminist values. The passive, self-effacing, exotic China doll needs to be replaced by the Woman Warrior image, a classic in Chinese mythology. A look at the evolution of women's roles in China, and the influence of Taoist as well as Confucian philosophy, is important to properly anchor

Jean Lau Chin, EdD, ABPP, was former Systemwide Dean, California School of Professional Psychology at Alliant International University. She is currently Dean, Gordon F. Derner Institute of Advanced Psychological Studies at Adelphi University.

Address correspondence to: Jean Lau Chin, Dean, Derner Institute, Adelphi University, P.O. Box 701, Garden City, NY 11530-0701 USA (E-mail: chin@adelphi.edu).

[Haworth co-indexing entry note]: "Psychotherapy for Asian American Woman Warriors." Chin, Jean Lau. Co-published simultaneously in *Women & Therapy* (The Haworth Press, Inc.) Vol. 30, No. 3/4, 2007, pp. 7-16; and: *Feminist Reflections on Growth and Transformation: Asian American Women in Therapy* (ed: Debra M. Kawahara, and Oliva M. Espín) The Haworth Press, Inc., 2007, pp. 7-16. Single or multiple copies of this article are available for a fee from The Haworth Document Delivery Service [1-800-HAWORTH, 9:00 a.m. - 5:00 p.m. (EST). E-mail address: docdelivery@haworthpress.com].

Available online at http://wt.haworthpress.com

doi:10.1300/J015v30n03_02

empowering roles for women to be supported in psychotherapy.
doi:10.1300/J015v30n03_02 *[Article copies available for a fee from The Haworth Document Delivery Service: 1-800-HAWORTH. E-mail address: <docdelivery@haworthpress.com> Website: <http://www.HaworthPress.com>*

KEYWORDS. Chinese American families, Chinese American women, storytelling, mythology

If we are to integrate multiculturalism and feminism for Chinese American women, we need to look at the images they conjure up. This is often through the media and literature. Negative stereotypes from the exotic China doll to the passive, self-effacing, obedient wife reflect the extremes of what Westerners would like to believe of the Asian American woman. These images become that of the Dragon Lady when she becomes assertive and dominant. One prominent image and classic Chinese story, that is more empowering, is that of *Hua Muk Lan* or the Woman Warrior. A view of the images and roles of Chinese women throughout history is revealing in identifying principles and strategies for psychotherapy with Asian American women.

THE WOMAN WARRIOR

While the image of Asian American women as *The Woman Warrior* has become popularized for Westerners through Maxine Hong Kingston's now classic book, and later by Disney in the movie *Mulan,* these westernized images of Asian American women derive from the classic Chinese story of *Hua Muk Lan*. Their differences reflect the evolution of the image contextualized by the perspective of the writer.

Hua Muk Lan, or the Woman Warrior as she is called in the West, is the heroine of the *Five Dynasties* (420-588), one of the most celebrated classics in the Chinese culture. This is a story of a young woman who loved and revered her aging father so much that when her aging father was called to battle, she goes in his place disguised as a man. For twelve years, she distinguishes herself in military battle as a warrior and leads the army to victory. She develops a friendship with a fellow military general whom she later marries after revealing her true self to him. She refuses further promotions, instead returns home to her parents and family, thereby fulfilling obligation to family.

A story celebrated by Chinese and Chinese American families to their children, this image is both empowering for women and illustrates the challenges they face in a society where males dominate. This classic story is paralleled by the triangular conflicts more common in Western fairy tales about girls and women. Snow White and Cinderella, for example, are like Hua Muk Lan in describing the journey of pubertal girls toward independence with a significant difference. Both need to be rescued by their prince charming while in conflict and competition with the wicked stepmother or queen. In Hua Muk Lan, the conflict and striving is played out outside the home, and emphasizes reunion between parent and child in the absence of intergenerational conflict.

Moreover, the mother is the bystander in contrast to the Western fairy tales where father is the bystander. The father's age prevents him from fulfilling his military obligations. Consequently, he approves of his daughter, Hua Muk Lan, to replace him in battle, i.e. independence and separation, in contrast to Western fairy tales that emphasize the pubertal girl's beauty as competitive and threatening in replacing the mother figure as queen. The child chooses to leave home, and does so to protect and rescue her father and family, and to fulfill her responsibility as the oldest sibling, representing some classic Chinese themes.

The theme of Hua Muk Lan celebrates the strength of women; military accomplishments are common themes in Chinese literature as studies of leadership, strategy, and intellect. The persistence of Hua Muk Lan as a popular story speaks to its appeal among the Chinese who love her intelligence, cleverness, and responsibility. It is notable, however, that her accomplishment and transformation can only be achieved in the guise of a man. Hua Muk Lan has become legendary and is loved particularly because she is discrepant with the image of women during Confucian times in China where military excellence, i.e., power, could only be achieved by a woman if she ceased to live as a woman.

Unlike Hua Muk Lan, other women in Chinese stories tend to achieve their power as concubines or courtesans since this was typically their only means to access positions of power. Most of these historic and legendary stories of other Chinese heroines were women of great character with stories of sacrifice and determination as they tried to fulfill their responsibilities, which were often conflicting (Yu, 1974). Typically, they achieved power and fame through their cleverness, responsibility, or prowess; in the end, they reunited with their families of origin as the final test of maturity.

Asian stories involving women commonly depict obligation as a developmental theme, which is achieved by the heroine after overcoming great odds. These themes contrast with the themes favored in Western fairy tales such as Snow White and Cinderella, where the heroine is more passive and receptive; her developmental task is to achieve sexual maturity and overcome narcissism before she can unite with the charming prince.

The images of women as wives in both Asian and Western mythology include that of temptress whose rise to power is shameless or complicit. However, as a mother in Asian mythology, she is powerful, benevolent, forgiving, nurturing, and a mentor. This contrasts with Western mythology where the theme is of mother as weak or wicked against a son who is competitive and aggressive.

WOMAN WARRIOR IMAGES IN HISTORY

While these themes and images of women whose primary assets are their beauty and wiliness are more common in both Western and Asian history, we need to question who writes that history and how it reflects the roles and images of women that men prefer to depict. Jones' study of female martial heritage found history replete with examples of Women Warriors across cultures, most of which were described in faint references (Jones, 1997). He describes:

> "the strength of women . . . is of a different kind: it is the ability to bear up under childbirth; it is nurturant depth; it is simple endurance of hardship . . . but the story of women's strength must not end there. . . . For women to deny their [warrior] tradition results in the loss of power that men freely employ." It is our social conditioning that results in dismissal of this role for women. "When females are not seen as warriors, their aspirations–the warrior prerogatives of power, choice, and control–become suspect as unnatural or unwomanlike." (p. xxi)

In looking at myths through the ages (Bierlein, 1994), Bachofen, a Swiss scholar of the Greek classics, came to the conclusion that there were three clear stages in early European culture. The first was a barbaric stage; this was followed by a matriarchy that, in turn, was supplanted by patriarchy. In the barbaric stage, neither male nor female were dominant in society resulting in widespread sexual promiscuity when children did not know their fathers, women were defenseless, and family life was virtually nonexistent. Aphrodite, the Greek goddess of love, characterized this period. . . . Next, women banded together for their own defense, leading to the development of a matriarchal society which is reflected in the Greek myths of Amazons and fierce woman warriors.

Bachofen's theory about European culture has its parallel in Chinese history and Asian culture where, according to Kristeva (1986), a matriarchy derived from peasant customs preceded the patriarchal Confucian family in China. A revolution in the rules of kinship took place in China, and can be traced to sometime around 1000 BC. While this happened similarly in the Mediterranean area, in China it was marked by the preservation of more elements from the earlier matriarchal model. Kristeva hypothesizes that this was due to the extraordinarily advanced development of the matrilineal family in China. A Chinese myth speaks to the existence of this age. The world is made habitable by Yu the Great (2198 BC), who organizes the lands and waters by causing the Yellow River to flow when he opens The Dragon's Gate; but first, he turns his wife to stone. His legendary creation dance imitated a feminine form as a symbol of political authority; when he is caught dancing by his wife, he kills her thus representing the sacrifice of the opposite sex to obtain this power. This sets the stage for patrilineal descent as monarchies are since passed from father to son, and forms the basis for Confucianism and the five rules of social order.

TAOISM AND BUDDHISM: EQUALITY OF THE SEXES AND MALE DOMINANCE

Confucianism is familiar to most Westerners and represents the prevalence of male dominance in Chinese society. Many use it to illustrate how Chinese American women are backward compared to Western women; i.e., why don't they stand up to their men? Why are they not more involved with the women's movement? Few are aware of the Taoist movement in China with its emphasis on the equality of the sexes, and how Chinese women through the ages have embraced issues of women empowerment through the Confucian era and during the Communist era in China.

Veneration for the mother is found throughout Chinese history in the ideologies of Buddhism and Taoism, which opposed itself to Confucianism and fostered many protests to the social order. The Book of Mountains and Sea (from the Taoist religion) has the story of the Queen Mother of the West, Hsi Wang Mu. She lives in a palace on a mythical jade mountain in the West. She was originally a monster with a human face, tiger's teeth, and a leopard's tail. But in Taoist legends, she became a beautiful goddess, quintessentially female, embodying the principle of yin. A peach tree, which blooms only once every three thousand years on the Queen Mother's birthday, grows there; those who eat its fruit gain immortality. It is at her birthday banquet that the legendary character, Monkey, stole a peach of immortality and was banished from heaven (Scott, 1980, p. 28).

Chinese Buddhism, in turn, has the goddess Kuan Yin, whose cult equals and sometimes surpasses that of Buddha himself. Kuan Yin, the Goddess of Mercy, on entering heaven is said to have paused to listen to the cry of the world, reflected in her name. A story placed in 7th century BC speaks of the daughter of a ruler who refused to marry according to the wishes of her parents, but was determined to enter a nunnery and devote her life to the poor and the sick (Scott, 1980, p. 38). Buddhism and Taoism in Confucian China were often a refuge for women since they acknowledged their equality with men. At the same time, these religions represented the contrasts between the peasants and nobility, and between men and women.

Confucianism emphasized the importance of the father-son relationships, probably dictated by economic reasons unlike the emotional bonds emphasized by mother-son relationships. Given the growing importance of agrarian society in feudal China prior to the Republic of China, Confucian times required a commitment of time and physical strength that mothers could not furnish. The feudal family followed Confucian tradition and teachings. Many of the early Toisanese immigrants to the U.S. were raised in a Confucian society, and it is these characteristics that are most known in the West as Chinese culture. The family was essentially an economic unit in which males were dominant. Continuity was ensured and marked by the son's reverence for the father, and his role as the heir apparent to ancestral line. There was an emphasis on a submissive attitude toward authority in the family or in government. Women and children were the ones over whom authority was exercised. Males were given the privilege of multiple wives, a demonstration of their wealth and social status. This, too, was hierarchical and collective. The only true mother was the first wife; all others were considered concubines with greater value if they produced sons. The children of all the wives belonged to the first wife or Dai Ma (Eldest Mother). The power in the family rested with the father, eldest son, and grandmother or eldest mother (Kristeva, 1986, p. 80).

A familiarity between father and daughter was more permissible in Confucian society, different from the distance and severity expected between father and son. While this gave women more room, it signified, at the same time, the total disregard of her in the social order where males reigned as the ancestors to be worshipped. Under Confucianism, women were destined only for housework and reproduction. In the words of several Confucianists, Yang Chen of the Han dynasty says, "If women are given work that requires contact with the outside, they will sow disorder and confusion throughout the Empire." Sima Guang of the Song dynasty says, "Give a woman an education and all you will get from her is boredom and complaints" (Kristeva, 1986, p. 76). The domination of women, in the words of these scholars, suggests the need to suppress the striving of women.

The Taoist tradition, on the other hand, never ceased to fight the Confucian paternalistic hierarchy. Women in China embraced Taoism as a religion because it emphasized the equality of women with men. Westerners often fail to realize this ambivalence and parallel challenge to Confucian emphasis on paternalism and male dominance in Asian cultures, or how the growth of Taoism in China paralleled some of the pioneer days and women's rights movement in America.

A frequent theme in Chinese history is that of the worthy Chinese woman, who braves death by letting herself be killed without flinching before the enemy or by committing suicide to facilitate the patriotic or revolutionary task of her husband or her clan as illustrated in The Guwen, a collection of classical texts (Kristeva, 1986, p. 94). This theme is also not uncommon among women and minorities in the U.S. where there is often the need to prove oneself by working twice as hard.

EVOLUTION OF WOMEN'S ROLES IN CHINA

A Ch'ing dynasty novel, *Flowers in the Mirror* (18th century), is both a fantasy and social satire on the plight of women. The author, believing in equal opportunity for men and women, sets the novel during the reign of Empress Wu who usurped the throne from her son in the early T'ang dynasty (604-705). As punishment for disobeying a decree, Tang Ao is dismissed from his scholarly rank, and forsakes the world for a long journey in search of immortality. Not unlike *Gulliver's Travels*, he passes through many fantastic lands where everything is strange, and comes to the Country of Women where it is the women who are talented and pass the imperial examinations while the men stay at home.

In Communist China, the heroine martyr was often celebrated as one who commits suicide as a means for young rebellion among young females. Having committed themselves to far-reaching ideals of emancipation in Communist China, many found no concrete means of realizing them such that Mao Tse Tung wrote:

> He who commits suicide is not motivated by a desire for death . . . most emphatic demonstration of the will to live. The reason why people commit suicide in a society is that the society has seized their hopes and brutally crushed them. . . . (Kristeva, 1986, p. 110)

In contemporary China, the Bourgeois Revolution of 1912 and the May 4th Movement of 1919 marked significant moments of the Women's Movement in China with threats to the Chinese family and patriarchy (Kristeva, 1986, p. 97; Barlow & Bjorge, 1989). This was represented particularly in the writings of Ding Ling, as well as other feminist writers from the early 20th century, who wrote of their plight and strivings to be liberated as intellectual equals with men. An interesting note is how Chinese women are perceived by Westerners as behind Western women in the women's movement when, in fact, the height of intellectual and political movements in China occurred well before its zenith in America.

EVOLUTION OF THE CHINESE WOMAN WARRIOR IMAGE

Ang Lee's movie, *Crouching Tiger, Hidden Dragon*, is a contemporary movie creating legend and myth based on Chinese culture set in the 19th century. Unlike classic Asian myths, the main protagonists are female. Yet, like many Asian classics, the outcome of this contemporary movie has the main protagonists dying or committing suicide and the lovers' union ending in tragedy. However, it is different from the classical hero's journey that is typically male and analogous as a rite of passage. Ang Lee transforms this movie into a feminine tale of self-discovery. Therefore, it is both classic and feminist (Simpson, 2001).

The ancient sword of legendary warrior, Li Mu Bai (the male hero and mentor) is stolen. In seeking enlightenment, he gave up his sword and entrusted it to his female warrior ally, Shu Lien, to take it to Governor Yu in Beijing for safekeeping. Shu Lien, the main female hero, arrives in Beijing and observes two young girls entertaining on the street. She is disdainful because she views these girls as slaves; yet, she too is trapped by her fate to remain a warrior. Each of the main characters has a journey toward self-discovery. The sword is stolen by the trickster Princess Jen, and protected by Jade Fox, the shadowy nemesis who killed Li Mu Bai's mentor. Li Mu Bai is forced to return the sword after it is stolen because he wants to avenge his mentor's death.

The dragon characteristics of Jen are hidden when she is behaving as the aristocratic princess; her impatience to reveal her hidden self and power reflects her youth. Classic myths and legends usually portrayed male and female characteristics rather dichotomously. Women needed to disguise themselves as men if they were to behave in a warrior-like fashion as in the Woman Warrior. This atypical portrayal of gender roles in the characters of Li Shen and Jen relies on classic Asian symbols as well as symbols from other cultures to create a legend about character transformation and the journey of enlightenment which makes *Crouching Tiger, Hidden Dragon* contemporary, relevant, and appealing.

IMPLICATIONS FOR PSYCHOTHERAPY

In reviewing these historic and legendary images and stories depicting the role of Chinese women as women warriors, we can see both the evolution of these roles, and the importance of contextualized images that need to be considered in today's context when working with Asian American women in psychotherapy. First, there is the need to challenge the negative and stereotypic images without obliterating the cultural values that underlie their genesis. Second, there is a need to promote more empowering images of the Woman Warrior without promoting the wanton use of aggression. Third, therapists need to draw from history and culture that include both the importance of cultural values and women's roles, while not rooting the therapy in Western assumptions nor in Asian contexts that are no longer meaningful to the contemporary Asian American woman. Lastly, the use of story by therapists in encouraging clients to create their family legends can be empowering as they help clients toward transformation and self-discovery (Chin, 2004).

For example, male dominant societies are prominent in both Western and Asian cultures as were the movements for female empowerment and gender equality. A comparative strategy to urge Asian American women to be more like their Western sisters is neither culturally competent nor feminist. Assertiveness training, commonly used as a strategy for teaching women to speak up and establish their voices, may not be appropriate for Asian American women if it fails to take into consideration the cultural strengths and differential ways of demonstrating assertiveness. While an understanding of the cultural roots and history of one's client is essential, therapists need to transcend their stereotypic images and contextualized roles in interpreting the stories that Asian American women bring to therapy. Lastly, the review of stories illustrates how images of Asian women will be influenced by the writer's perspective; similarly, a therapist's perspective too will be influenced by his/her own cultural perspective and counter-transference issues.

REFERENCES

Barlow, T. E., & Bjorge, G. J. (Eds.) (1989). *I myself am a woman. Selected writings of Ding Ling*. Boston: Beacon Press.

Bierlein, J. F. (1994). *Parallel myths.* New York: Ballantine Books.

Chin, J. L. (2004). *Learning from my mother's voice: Family legend and Chinese American immigration.* New York: TC Press.

Jones, D. (1997). *Women warriors: A history.* Dulles, VA: Brassey's.

Kingston, M. H. (1989). *The Woman Warrior: Memoirs of a girlhood among ghosts.* New York: Random House.

Kristeva, J. (1986). *About Chinese women.* New York: Marion Boyars.

Scott, D. H. (1980). *Chinese popular literature and the child.* Chicago: American Library Association.

Simpson, C. S. (2001, March 23). Crouching Tiger: The rebirth of myth. *The Chronicle of Higher Education*, p. B19.

Yu, L. (1974). *Chinese women in history and legend.* New York: A.R.T.S.

doi:10.1300/J015v30n03_02

"Making a Difference": Asian American Women Leaders

Debra M. Kawahara

SUMMARY. This paper attempts to explore the intersection of Asian American culture and gender on leadership. This qualitative study examined the lives of two Asian American women leaders, building on a previous study conducted by Kawahara, Esnil, and Hsu (in press). Six themes from the previous study are found as well as two new themes which emerged from the two interviews. Limitations of current psychological theories on intersecting identities are discussed. doi:10.1300/J015v30n03_03

KEYWORDS. Asian American, women, leadership, feminism, multiculturalism

---

Debra M. Kawahara, PhD, is Assistant Professor in Clinical Psychology, California School of Professional Psychology at Alliant International University.

Address correspondence to: Debra M. Kawahara, California School of Professional Psychology, Alliant International University, 10455 Pomerado Road, San Diego, CA 92131-1799 USA (E-mail: dkawahara@alliant.edu).

[Haworth co-indexing entry note]: " 'Making a Difference': Asian American Women Leaders." Kawahara, Debra M. Co-published simultaneously in *Women & Therapy* (The Haworth Press, Inc.) Vol. 30, No. 3/4, 2007, pp. 17-33; and: *Feminist Reflections on Growth and Transformation: Asian American Women in Therapy* (ed: Debra M. Kawahara, and Oliva M. Espín) The Haworth Press, Inc., 2007, pp. 17-33. Single or multiple copies of this article are available for a fee from The Haworth Document Delivery Service [1-800-HAWORTH, 9:00 a.m. - 5:00 p.m. (EST). E-mail address: docdelivery@haworthpress.com].

Available online at http://wt.haworthpress.com

doi:10.1300/J015v30n03_03

Little scholarship exists regarding the experiences of Asian American women compared to that of European American women (Comas-Diaz & Greene, 1994; Chin, 2000). What is available has focused on topics such as familial roles and relationships, cultural values, attitudes and beliefs. Unfortunately, some popular literature and media continue to perpetuate the stereotypes of Asian American women as passive, exotic, or victims of a patriarchal "traditional" Asian culture (Espiritu, 1997). As a result, the racialization of Asian womanhood blends racism and sexism by presenting Asian and Asian American women as stereotypically feminine, thus upholding white superiority. Research on leadership among Asian American women is even more sparse than the general descriptive literature on Asian American community and families. Despite the continued growth of the Asian American population and the increasing diversity within this group, the rising visibility of advocacy and activism among Asian American women leaders is seldom addressed.

This article is a continuation of a previously published research project (Kawahara, Esnil, & Hsu, in press) aimed at exploring the intersection of Asian American culture and gender on leadership. The project was prompted by Dr. Jean Lau Chin's presidential initiative for the American Psychological Association's Society for the Psychology of Women in 2002. A primary goal of her initiative was to examine how women lead and the ways that multiple intersections of identities (race, ethnicity, gender, class, and profession) influence leadership styles. Internet-based websites for 15 different topics were created to facilitate dialogue on diversity, collaboration, and leadership. The overall goal was to build upon Norine Johnson's book *Shaping the Future of Feminist Psychology* and to draw from a variety of viewpoints, models, and perspectives in order to promote diversity and feminist leadership.

In following these web-based dialogues, our interests in Asian American women and leadership peaked. We wanted to further understand the complex interactions of gender and race in the experiences of Asian American women leaders. A qualitative interview study seemed like an excellent method to understand this phenomenon where there is very little scholarship and knowledge. Core feminist concepts of resiliency and strength, empowerment, personal reflexivity, power relations, and connectedness are the underlying values that we used to guide our understanding and exploration of the phenomenon. Also, we intentionally attempted to include diverse Asian ethnicities and areas of interests to honor these women's subjectivities given the heterogeneity of Asian American women. The women interviewed were identified as high-achieving Asian American women leaders in their particular field or profession. The overall goal of the research project was to examine these women's paths to leadership and illuminate the context of both gender and race to understand leadership from a feminist perspective. Hopefully, this is an important step in transforming psychology to include diverse voices in developing a vision for the future.

HISTORICAL BACKGROUND OF ASIAN AMERICAN WOMEN

Immigration Patterns

As noted by Mazumdar (2003), immigration patterns of Asian American women were similar to the immigrant women from Europe. Many of the women served domestic roles in the 1800s and early 1900s, while the men became sojourners to fill the labor needs of the global economy. However, unlike the European women, anti-miscegenation and exclusion laws prevented Asian American women from immigrating to the U.S. in larger numbers and actually suppressed the number of Asian women immigrants as compared to Asian men, actually as recently as indicated by the 1970 U.S. census (Bradshaw, 1994).

The initial wave of immigration to the U.S. in the mid-1800s included Chinese women. Many were given false promises of the riches in the new land, were sold by their family, or kidnapped to work as prostitutes. Because of the growing anti-Asian sentiment and the immorality of the Chinese "bachelor society," the larger society felt justified in passing laws which limited immigration and this atmosphere discouraged other Chinese women, such as wives, daughters, and mothers of the men sojourners, to make the move. The initial wave was then followed by a wave of Japanese and Korean women before 1924. However, this second wave of immigration was curtailed by the Gentleman's Agreement in 1907 that consisted of a quota of immigrants per country and significantly restricted immigration of Japanese and Korean women, followed by the 1924 Immigration Act that completely ended immigration for many Asian groups. Despite these measures, a large influx of Korean women entered the U.S. after the Korean War (1950-1965). Additionally, another immigrant group of women, primarily Japanese, became wives of military personnel during the U.S. involvement in the Pacific between 1947 and 1977 and, thus, gained entry to the U.S. (Bradshaw, 1994).

The next wave of immigration came after the Immigration Act of 1965 that eased restrictions on Asian immigration. Women from China, Korea, the Philippines, South Asia, and Southeast Asia immigrated in large numbers and were more educated than their predecessors (Bradshaw, 1994). For example, Filipina and Southeast Asian women attained the highest educational levels statistically among all Asian immigrant groups (Bradshaw, 1994).

These waves of immigration patterns seemed to have implications for Asian American women leaders. For the study, a valiant attempt was made to be inclusive of diverse Asian ethnicities; however, the complete purposive interview sample was composed of five Chinese and five Japanese women with Filipinas following as the next most represented ethnicity with three women. It was surmised that the resulting sample was a reflection of the immigration patterns and that those women in ethnic groups with longer histories in the U.S. were allowed more time and resources to establish and make inroads into the larger U.S. society.

UNDERSTANDING THE SUBJECTIVITIES OF RACE AND GENDER

The intersection of race and gender is of particular interest in the lived experiences of these Asian American women leaders because each represents an oppressive force in society. Both dimensions of identity are often a focal point of identity development because of the need to integrate oppressed aspects of oneself into one's holistic identity. As such, leadership in different contexts would seem to be influenced by the development of one's biculturalism and gender identity.

Biculturalism

The negotiating of different cultures is often referred to as biculturalism, meaning that Asian American women have two internalized cultures that guide their thoughts, perceptions, and feelings (LaFromboise, Coleman, & Gerton, 1993; Phinney & Devich-Navarro, 1997). One is the woman's Asian culture and the other is the dominant American culture. Whether these women are able to do this effectively will depend on their bicultural efficacy. *Bicultural efficacy* is defined as the ability to develop and maintain interpersonal relations within two groups without relinquishing one's cultural identity (LaFromboise et al., 1993). In such situations, it is believed that the person's bicultural competence will assist her in building and maintaining support networks in the different contexts while also providing support when either group rejects her or when she is developing competence in one group.

Asian American women are faced with the task of developing competency in a majority cultural setting in which they are a minority, while maintaining their cultural connections to one another. Ideally, the bicultural individual develops the skills and abilities to be competent in a second culture without losing that same competence in the culture of origin. Ultimately, successful bicultural individuals have a sense of psychological well-being as well as mastery in their social, work, and family environments.

Feminist Identity Development

Another major identity dimension for Asian American women is gender. Parallel to the implications of race on her ability to function in the world, the implications of gender have to be negotiated and worked through given the patriarchal structure embedded in both U.S. and Asian societies. Gender-based identity development models assist in understanding the process of consciousness about the subjugation of women in society and the development of a feminist identity.

Downing and Roush (1985) developed a feminist identity model based on W. E. Cross's 1971 view of the development of African American identity. It is a five-stage model that includes (1) passive acceptance; (2) revelation; (3) embeddedness-emanation; (4) synthesis; and (5) active commitment. The stages of the model are seen as more cyclical than linear in nature in that a person can return to a previous stage after reaching a higher stage because of life circumstances or experiences.

The first stage of passive acceptance is where the female accepts traditional gender roles, sees males as advantageous to her, and considers men to be superior to women. This changes in the second stage of revelation. At this point, sexist acts become evident and the individual becomes aware of the prejudice, becomes angry, and feels guilty for the lack of awareness in the previous stage. There is intense questioning of one's beliefs and the woman often holds dichotomous views of men as bad and women as good. The third stage is embeddedness-emanation. The woman at this stage forms close emotional relationships and connectedness with other women. As her feminist identity solidifies, she begins to view men in a more relativistic than dualistic manner. Synthesis occurs when the woman develops a positive feminist identity and no longer considers sexism as the only cause for all social and personal problems, but also considers other causal factors. This is marked by a transcendence of gender roles in which men are evaluated on an individual basis as opposed to a group basis. In the last stage of active commitment, the woman is firmly grounded in her feminist identity and makes a commitment to making societal changes.

Although the psychological aspects of race and gender were presented separately, the dynamic and complex interplay of these dimensions into one's identity cannot be dismissed or ignored. The aforementioned concepts are understood as singular dimensions and lack the integration of the dualism between race and gender among all the other identity dimensions that define these women. This has been and continues to be a major criticism of the stage-like models of identity development and has prompted the movement toward more comprehensive models that embrace the multiple subjectivities of people.

INTERVIEW STUDY

The original study had 12 women participants who were of Asian descent. A purposive sample of diverse Asian ethnicities and professions among the women was obtained. Each of the women selected were considered to be high achievers as well as leaders in their respective field or profession, all within a U.S. context. This study focused on two women who were of Asian descent, specifically Japanese American, and not included in the original study. Table 1 shows demographic characteristics of all the women in the entire sample with the two women in this study at the bottom of the table.

The original sample consisted of five Chinese American women, three Filipinas, two Japanese American women, one South Asian Indian woman, and one biracial woman (Japanese-African American). The following professions were represented: educational administrator, entrepreneur, judge, magazine editor and founder, musician/artist, psychologist, state legislator, public policy administrator, and university professor. In this study, the professions of the two Japanese American women participants are CEO/hospital administrator (retired) and Ordained Minister.

Procedures for all the women were the same. Each of the women were interviewed either in-person or by phone. An interview guide consisting of three questions was developed and later elaborated to five questions by the research team from the first study. However,

TABLE 1. Interviewee Demographics

Interviewee Name*	Ethnicity	National Origin	Profession	Educational Level
Donna Tsui	Chinese American	U.S.	Public policy administrator	Masters
Julianna Tang	Chinese American	U.S.	Musician/artist	Unknown
Wendy Chen	Chinese American	U.S.	University administrator	Ed.D.
Diane Liu	Chinese American	U.S.	University administrator	Ed.D.
Sharon Lee	Chinese American	U.S.	State legislator	Ph.D.
Jordan Nabe	Filipina	Philippines	Entrepreneur	Some College
Olivia Ramirez	Filipina	U.S.	Director of university-based women's health program	Ph.D.
Ling Marsela	Filipina	Philippines	Magazine editor and founder	M.A
Tammie Fuji	Japanese	Japan	Psychologist	Ph.D.
Lynn Takasaki	Japanese American	U.S.	Judge	J.D.
Katherine Bell	Japanese-African American	U.S.	College administrator	Ph.D.
Sikha Mishra	South Asian	India	University professor	Ph.D.
Ramona Kimura McAllister	Japanese American	U.S.	Ordained Minister	M. Div.
Keiko Bouchler	Japanese American	U.S.	CEO/administrator of university hospital (Retired)	M.A.

*Actual names have been changed to pseudonyms.

interviews went beyond the areas of the interview guide depending on the interviewee's response. We utilized various avenues to recruit participants for the research study. Some of the women were professional contacts through our own network, whereas others were sought out because of their known status and work in their communities, or were referred by women who participated in the study.

Once a woman was identified, one of us contacted her and scheduled an appointment if she agreed to participate. The two women in this study were interviewed by the author of this article. One of the interviews lasted three hours and the other interview was two hours in length. The interview was audiotaped and the interviewer kept journal notes to document observations and thoughts about the interview. For the first study, the interviews were transcribed for analysis. We then read all the transcripts numerous times and discussed the themes and dynamics delineated from the interviews. There were six themes that emerged from the 12 women in the first study. They were: knowing thyself and doing something you believe in; having a vision and inspiring others to work on that vision; utilizing a relational and collaborative leadership style; taking on challenges, struggles, and conflicts; displaying dominant culture efficacy and biculturalism; and having support and encouragement.

RESULTS

In the second study, I followed the procedures outlined above and then corroborated the data from the transcripts with the previous study's results (for more information regarding the first study, refer to Kawahara, Esnil, & Hsu, in press). The first study's themes were further supported by the two women's interviews as well as two additional themes that emerged which included familial and childhood influences as well as a Christian influence.

Ebb and Flow of Life

Similar to the eight women in the first study who discussed ebb and flow of life, both of the women in this study were guided by their life situations and experiences as well as by the social milieu of the time. Their life stage and cohort seemed to shape what they valued and believed and allowed them to shift when the situation changed. Unlike a more masculine approach of strategically planning one's career, the women found a more emergent, evolving process that weaved together their self-knowledge, growth, interests, and experiences.

> I didn't say I wanted to be a minister, you know like some people when they're really young, they want to do that. . . . It really was circumstances I think that created the opportunities for me. . . . (Ramona, Ordained Minister)

> The big thing which is a stumbling block for me is when kids ask me how did you decide, how did you mold your career? And the answer is that I just went from one thing to another. . . . (Keiko, CEO/hospital administrator)

Furthermore, Ramona and Keiko, like the women in the first study, were more often asked and/or encouraged to apply to leadership and/or management positions because others recognized their superior work and abilities as opposed to them actively seeking out a higher position or status. However, the women had to be willing to apply and take on the responsibilities of the position once it was presented.

> So it was a perfect opportunity, I needed to get out before it got tainted with all that and so it was good for me, and it turned out just by luck and happenstance that Mike got, number one got named CEO, actually he came to talk to me as soon as my other boss got fired, he felt really bad about it and he said well come and work in [*city*], and I said you don't really have a job, he said you don't really have a job there. . . . So I did get the job. (Keiko, CEO/hospital administrator)

> And then we had the national conference, and then they pick of 135 churches and they pick seven. So I was chosen for those things within the conference really early on in my ministry. So I don't know, sometimes I'm even surprised when I get chosen for things. Like when I went to Chicago I was chosen for the national moderator. (Ramona, Ordained Minister)

Having a Vision and Inspiring Others to Work on the Vision

Again, a prominent theme among the women was the belief that a leader has to have a vision and be able to inspire others to follow and act on the vision. Additionally, the leader has to exude excitement and enthusiasm about the vision and rally others' assistance to make it a reality.

> But, I think basically they're just very simple, the ability to get people to work together to achieve a common goal, very simple, whether it's just you and you're talking your younger sister into doing something stupid, or you know, it's just the ability to get folks to do whatever needs to be done to achieve whatever goals

> and the bigger the number of people, the larger the group, the greater the goal, the more leadership is needed. . . . (Keiko, CEO/hospital administrator)

> I said, what now, God tells you something, what is the next step? [Robert said] You need to tell your Board of Trustees. . . . Yeah, just share it with them. Well I shouldn't be afraid to present this to them. It was really God's will, they're going to receive the same thing. So I brought it to the Board of Trustees, I had a vision, I had a vision workshop first. . . . I presented the ideas to the trustees. . . . So this group is really wonderful. Everything I presented to them, they accepted. (Ramona, Ordained Minister)

Similar to seven women in the first study, the two women in this study felt a deep sense of responsibility and commitment to "make a difference." The impact of their work was to make things better and seemed to go beyond their own immediate self-interests.

> Just being the kind of person I am, whatever I was in, I wanted to do the best, to do the best, I wanted to make a difference. If I was gonna be in that position, I wanted to make a difference. I just didn't want to be, you know, mediocre. (Ramona, Ordained Minister)

Relational and Collaborative Leadership Style

Related to the leader's values, vision, and inspiration to others, these two women, like eight of the women in the previous study, used a more decentralized and participatory leadership style. The women recognized the strengths of others, empowered others by sharing power, and were willing to learn, work hard, and share through the process. Also, relationships among the group members were valued as much as achieving the working goals.

> I think that you really have to love your people. It's as if they know that you love them, they go the extra mile for you. Like, years ago, I had this secretary from South Carolina, she said you're the only boss I had that I can pray with [in the corporate world]. (Ramona, Ordained Minister)

> I just knew I wasn't the best person to be the one to step in. I wouldn't pay the right kind of attention so they would feel valued

> so it was important for me to have a lieutenant who reached the gap so to speak and she was perfect because I wanted to get a lot of progress made. . . . She just did extraordinary kind of things . . . the facts spoke for themselves, the ladies loved her, she got the job done, my end goals were taken care of in spite of my goals which could have been from these ladies' point of view a very, very adversarial thing to do where she accomplished all that. (Keiko, CEO/hospital administrator)

Taking on Challenges, Struggles, and Conflicts

As part of being a leader, the women had to be willing to step up when an opportunity arose or a problem was seen and take action. This meant that not only could the women identify problems or needs, but they also had to be willing to do something about it.

> I had a real run in with this person who I picked as chairperson. And he got into this real macho male ego thing. It was more important for him to impress other men of the church than to follow guidelines that I had. And he made a really sarcastic remark about "I don't have to listen to you." I just listened and said, "You know, [*name*], I am the pastor of this church. And you know I get a lot of my direction from God, and so in other words, you're saying we don't count." . . . About a month, oh, he said he was gonna quit then. But I really didn't want him to quit. So I let him think about it for a week . . . I said I really feel that God calls us to a certain place. No matter what God challenges us. And then he apologized and said I'll support you and I'll stay on. (Ramona, Ordained Minister)

Obtaining and honing leadership skills such as communication and public speaking, listening, organizing, fundraising, educating, conflict resolution, and networking were essential for these women to be effective as leaders.

> I could take advantage of everything I was learning about [in the graduate healthcare program] and it truly helped me organize my thought processes about what's going on in organizations. I mean really you get out there, you jump into an organization, the bigger it is, the worse it is and what you see is a bunch of motion, but in-

> stead, you read the motion. It's repetitive . . . and actually the whole process of labeling and understanding concepts brings to you a knowledge that you use for the rest of your life . . . to then know how do I want to address it, what are the outcomes, the potential options I have here. (Keiko, CEO/hospital administrator)

Dominant Culture Efficacy and Biculturalism

As in the first study, both of the women focused on the necessity to work and be visible in multiple cultural settings, particularly within the dominant culture. What was remarkable was that these women did not believe that being an Asian American woman was something that held them back or was a detriment.

> Never, no, I can honestly look at you and say it never affected me cause I never defined myself as a female administrator of Asian persuasion, I mean I was just me. (Keiko, CEO/hospital administrator)

> I know years ago when I was in politics, someone asked the question about how Asian women felt that they were at a disadvantage of being electable because they were Asian. And I said I really disagree with that. Your Asian persona should not be a detriment, because if you're hardworking, if you like people, if you are willing to go that extra mile, your race shouldn't be a barrier. And I think we see that in all people. (Ramona, Ordained Minister)

Support and Freedom

In the first study, 11 out of the 12 women discussed the importance of others for support, guidance, and mentoring. Whether it was within their families or in persons outside familial lines, the women found people who believed in them, who they could turn to for advice, and who supported them through the setbacks and difficulties. In addition to the support and encouragement, the two women in this study also emphasized the importance of the freedom to be who they are and to be able to do what was needed.

> You know it wasn't anything we ever discussed and stuff so it was just that way but it was very important . . . the big thing is the free-

> dom to do what I thought needed to be done and secondly always having him (partner) there to be supportive. That was a huge huge thing. (Keiko, CEO/hospital administrator)

> But I think one of the reasons too about being raised by Japanese in Hawaii. And so, we didn't have any kind of civilized tension. Maybe other Asians, Japanese might have. We're not here on the mainland. You know because in Hawaii we didn't have that. So we felt that freedom to be who we are. (Ramona, Ordained Minister)

Familial and Childhood Influences

In both women, their families appeared to have a significant impact on who they became and who they are today. Both came from larger close-knit families. One came from a family of seven children and the other came from a family of six children. Both seemed to have older sibling(s) that they admired or wanted to be like and were emotionally close to. In addition, each had a parent who seemed to possess more extraverted characteristics such that their parent's persona would counter stereotypes typically held about Asian men and women.

> So usually you see Japanese meant to be real sweet and demure, but she [mom] wasn't. She was loud, she was boisterous. She was a tomboy, and she was extremely beautiful when she young. (Ramona, Ordained Minister)

> He [dad] was always a strong-minded person, he knew, a lot of self-confidence, knew what he wanted and he had a charismatic piece to him that was clear from people who knew him. And he had a clear influence on everybody and that influence I'd say for the most part was just a feeling of confidence. (Keiko, CEO/hospital administrator)

Christian Influence

Both women had Christian teachings in their childhood. In the case of Keiko, her mother identified as Catholic, even though the rest of the family was Buddhist. Keiko and her siblings attended Catholic school. For Ramona, her parents allowed her to become a Christian as a child. She describes her spiritual path as waxing and waning and eventually becoming her "calling."

> You know I never knew what call meant, but when God puts a call in your heart, you cannot escape it. And then you read the Bible, you read about people that God touch or call in their hearts, and they too cannot run away, you know? You always come back to it. So, you know, I had a shallow faith early in life, and through my hardships, I guess I just, you know, drew me closer to him. (Ramona, Ordained Minister)

DISCUSSION

As the project began, we knew many Asian American women and more specifically, Asian American women leaders, who do not fit the prescribed characteristics of the stereotypes of Asian American women as being passive, submissive, demure, exotic, and apolitical. Clearly, the Asian American women that I interviewed did not fit the stereotypes and characteristics often imposed on Asian American women, nor do they reflect the literature and media that portray them as objects/victims of external forces of prejudice and discrimination.

First, the women were active participants in their continual process of self-awareness. They seemed to have a clear sense of who they are, what they believe in, and where they want to go. They are agents of their own lives and provide direction for others. In effect, they determine their own destiny, creating paths for themselves and others. It is not to say that there are not contextual dynamics and issues such as oppression and prejudice that influence how the path is negotiated. Nonetheless, the women appear to take their evolving sense of self and find opportunities that allow themselves to engage in activities that are fulfilling. This foundation gives them direction and allows them to inspire and engage others in that direction because their actions are driven by their values and passion.

Interestingly, the women seemed to have a sense of responsibility to the larger group that motivates their actions. Consistent with the historical literature, much of the women's work and leadership involved making a difference in their communities and society-at-large. Advocacy and working toward social justice seemed to be important components of their vision. They could identify with those who were less visible, less heard, and less powerful in the system, and wanted to change it for the betterment of society.

To be leaders, the women learned new skills and faced challenges, struggles, and conflicts directly. Being communicative, managing conflicts, understanding organizational dynamics, and seeing the talents and strengths of others were abilities that the women developed and utilized to lead. In addition to these skills, the women recognized the need to be effective in interacting and working within the dominant culture. It seemed very important to neither perceive themselves as being at a disadvantage because they were Asian American women nor attribute any barriers or problems to their race or gender. They held a "can-do" attitude, no matter what obstacles or struggles confronted them and expected to work harder than the next person. Support, encouragement, and freedom from others assisted these women in facing the struggles, overcoming barriers, guiding them through the unknown, and providing them with a sense of belonging and acceptance to be themselves.

These actions suggested that these women used the values and behaviors of both the Asian and the dominant culture in order to achieve their goals. In fact, their actions are consistent with the literature on bicultural competence in LaFromboise et al.'s model. Moreover, these actions suggest that these women fit the latter stages of the feminist identity model.

Overall, the women's leadership style had a collectivistic view in both what they were doing and in the way that they lead. In both cases, a focus on the group rather than the individual, and relationships with others are primary. Learning, sharing, including, and working together through empowerment appears to be important to many of the women. This collectivistic view is consistent with both Asian American cultural values and feminist values. From the interviews, it could not be ascertained whether this group orientation derives from their Asian American cultural heritage, their feminist perspective, their disposition, or a combination of factors.

As the process of examining these women's stories unfolded, it became clear that there is multidimensionality and complexity that influence these women's lives throughout their whole being. It was not that they were Asian, or that they were women, or that they were an administrator or reverend that made them leaders. These multiple identity dimensions are intertwined with one another as well as with their unique life experiences. The experiences described by these women supported the assertion that it is impossible to examine one identity dimension at a time (e.g., race) separate from other dimensions (e.g, gender), hoping to somehow combine them to understand their intersections. Espin (2005) pointed out how this can manifest in the therapeutic relationship when the therapist's discomfort in not being able to "pin down" the client is more the problem in therapy than the client's multiple sense of identity.

Future psychological theories of women's identity development and clinical practice will need to integrate these multiple subjectivities and identity dimensions. These studies also demonstrate the need to develop new dynamic models to understand the intersections in their complexity and specificity. It seems that psychology is not yet at a place that understands identities that incorporate several crucial selves and internal contradictions (Espin, 2005).

For instance, I reviewed models of biculturalism and feminist identity development. The models offered explanations of a process and stages for a particular identity dimension. Yet, none of the models could fully capture the experiences being explored nor explain what was emerging from the women's interviews because the models compartmentalized and separated the dimensions. This finding is important for feminist practitioners to be aware of when clinically working with Asian American women. Overall, the models lacked sophistication for what I and the other research team members were attempting to understand. Theory building is a process and I do not believe that these models have completely outlived their descriptive utility. However, I believe that more elaborate models must take into account the interactions and integration of the multiple, diverse identity dimensions.

The purpose of this research was to continue to gain a better understanding of Asian American women leaders. The research is limited by several factors. First, we intentionally examined the two dimensions of race and gender. Certainly, there are many other dimensions such as socioeconomic class, religion, time period, geographical location, age, sexual orientation, disabilities, and motherhood status that influence the women and their leadership. Second, we chose to interview diverse Asian ethnic women. We know that there is much heterogeneity among Asian ethnic groups and believe that more specificity would come from investigating one Asian ethnic group, such as sampling only Filipina women. Third, we interviewed Asian women with diverse professions. Again, we believe the interviews would have been different if we interviewed women from the same profession. Fourth, we asked certain questions and interacted in certain ways with the interviewees because of who we are and where we are in our own developmental journeys. This definitely influenced how the women we interviewed responded and the outcome of the interview itself.

As in the first study, I believe that the opportunity to hear these women's stories and share them with others is a gift to be cherished. They are truly powerful women who are inspiring and motivating others. The women illuminate the agency in their lives and counter the stereotypes of the passive, submissive or exotic, sexualized Asian American woman. These interviews highlight the accomplishments by Asian American women that are often overlooked or invisible to others because of such stereotypes. Furthermore, these interviews illustrate the strength, resilience, intelligence, and competence of these powerful Asian American women leaders. For feminist practitioners, it is important to remember and emphasize these women and their work when working with other Asian American women in a clinical setting.

REFERENCES

Bradshaw, C. G. (1994). Asian and Asian American women: Historical and political considerations in psychotherapy. In L. Comas-Diaz & B. Greene (Eds.), *Women of color: Integrating ethnic and gender identities in psychotherapy* (pp. 72-113). New York: Guilford Press.

Chin, J. L. (Ed.) (2000). *Relationships among Asian American women.* Washington, DC: American Psychological Association.

Comas-Diaz, L., & Greene, B. (Eds.) (1994). *Women of color: Integrating ethnic and gender identities in psychotherapy.* New York: Guilford Press.

Downing, N., & Roush, K. (1985). From passive acceptance to active commitment: A model of feminist identity development for women. *The Counseling Psychologist, 13,* 695-709.

Espin, O. (2005, January). *The age of the cookie cutter has passed: Contradiction in identity at the core of therapeutic intervention.* Paper presented at the National Multicultural Conference and Summit, Los Angeles, CA.

Espiritu, Y. L. (1997). *Asian American women and men: Labor, laws, and love.* Thousand Oaks, CA: Sage Publications.

Kawahara, D. M., Esnil, E. M., & Hsu, J. (in press). Agency and empowerment of Asian American women leaders. In J. L. Chin, B. Lott, J. Rice, & J. Sanchez-Hucles (Eds.), *Feminist leadership: Visions and diverse voices.* Washington, DC: American Psychological Association.

LaFromboise, T., Coleman, H. L. K., & Gerton, J. (1993). Psychological impact of biculturalism: Evidence and theory. *Psychological Bulletin, 114,* 395-412.

Mazumdar, S. (2003). What happened to the women? Chinese and Indian male migration to the United States in global perspective. In S. Hune & G. M. Nomura (Eds.), *Asian/Pacific Islander American women: A historical anthology* (pp. 58-74). New York: New York University Press.

Phinney, J., & Devich-Navarro, M. (1997). Variations in bicultural identification among African-American and Mexican American adolescents. *Journal of Research on Adolescence, 7,* 918-927.

doi:10.1300/J015v30n03_03

CONSTRUCTION OF IDENTITY

Too Maternal and Not Womanly Enough: Asian-American Women's Gender Identity Conflict

Sung Ha Suh

SUMMARY. The paper discusses the unique challenges Asian-American women face in defining their gender identity. The variations between the views of Asian immigrant mothers and their daughters on their identity and roles as women reflect their respective socialization. Whereas the mothers have been socialized in traditional Confucian, gender-specific cultures wherein women are afforded fewer economic and social opportunities to develop as individuals, their daughters are immersed in American culture conducive to the development of gender ideals of personal autonomy, self-definition, and egalitarianism. The daughters' life experience and exposure to two distinct and often con-

Sung Ha Suh, PhD, is Assistant Professor in Counseling Psychology, John Jay College of Criminal Justice at The City University of New York.

Address correspondence to: Sung Ha Suh, PhD, Counseling Department, John Jay College of Criminal Justice, The City University of New York, 445 West 59th Street, New York, NY 10019 (E-mail: ssuh@jjay.cuny.edu).

[Haworth co-indexing entry note]: "Too Maternal and Not Womanly Enough: Asian-American Women's Gender Identity Conflict." Suh, Sung Ha. Co-published simultaneously in *Women & Therapy* (The Haworth Press, Inc.) Vol. 30, No. 3/4, 2007, pp. 35-50; and: *Feminist Reflections on Growth and Transformation: Asian American Women in Therapy* (ed: Debra M. Kawahara, and Oliva M. Espín) The Haworth Press, Inc., 2007, pp. 35-50. Single or multiple copies of this article are available for a fee from The Haworth Document Delivery Service [1-800-HAWORTH, 9:00 a.m. - 5:00 p.m. (EST). E-mail address: docdelivery@haworthpress.com].

Available online at http://wt.haworthpress.com

doi:10.1300/J015v30n03_04

flicting cultural orientations of female gender ideals enable them to broadly exercise their discretion in redefining and creating their own identity as a distinct group of women in the United States. Complications arising out of the daughters' inability to breach their Eastern heritage with mainstream ideals are discussed in the context of how they self-identify and are identified by their traditional culture and by mainstream society. doi:10.1300/J015v30n03_04 *[Article copies available for a fee from The Haworth Document Delivery Service: 1-800-HAWORTH. E-mail address: <docdelivery@haworthpress.com> Website: <http://www.HaworthPress.com>*

KEYWORDS. Asian-American women, female identity, mother-daughter relationship

Cross-cultural studies have addressed the ethnic identity conflicts experienced by the younger generation of Asian-Americans, but the unique challenges that Asian-American women encounter in defining their gender identity as a result of their exposure to distinct and often conflicting cultural gender ideologies have not received comparable attention. Studies of Asian-Americans' gender experience have explored gender-role attitudes. A vast majority of these studies indicates that Western cultures evince more egalitarian gender-based attitudes than Confucian Asian cultures (Williams & Best, 1990; Chang, 1999). The primary focus of these studies has been on comparing cross-cultural orientations and the collective experience of both men and women. However, the experiences of Asian-American women are qualitatively different from those of their male counterparts and their non-Asian female contemporaries precisely because their roles and status as women are characterized by mainstream assumptions and stereotypes of Asian-American women based on a well-defined set of traditional norms, expectations, and values. The primary basis of this paper is to give voice and visibility to the unique experiences and challenges that the younger generation of Asian-American women face upon recognizing that they can no longer be guided purely by traditions and experiences embodied in their mothers.

THE ROLE OF THE MOTHER-DAUGHTER RELATIONSHIP

Although a lot of people influence a daughter's conception of herself as a woman, the role of mother-daughter relationship is salient to understanding Asian-American daughters' gender identity conflicts. My interest in the female members of Asian ethnic families stems from the fact that historically, the central role for women in Confucian societies was largely confined to the domestic realm. At an early age, girls' socialization was steeped in filial obligations, feminine virtues, and domestic duties. Upon marriage, women were confined to the roles of childbearing, child rearing, and homemaking, whereas the public domain was sanctioned only for men. Although Asia has rapidly changed from a traditional to a modern society, traditional Confucian gender ideals remain deeply embedded in its social structure.

Asian-American women's conception of womanhood poses interesting challenges for Asian women because their migration and acculturation expose them to conflicting gender and social situations. The efforts to maintain a core family structure in a new and unfamiliar environment require all members of an immigrant household, regardless of gender, to adjust to their adopted culture by taking on new roles. However, the cultural shifts are much more compelling for the females than for the male members of an immigrant family because new gender ideologies that identify providers and authority figures based on capacity challenge the differential roles. Thus, the expectations for Asian-American sons to become the provider remain relatively the same, whereas, the expectations for the daughters to become wage earners and assume leadership positions are less common.

The greater transitions for the female members also yield greater generational disparity between the mothers and the daughters, which would not exist anywhere near to the same degree in their countries of origin. Even for second generation ethnic families in the U.S., traditional gender relations are characterized through their cultural lineage and reinforced by mainstream biases. The variance in the ways members of each generation are socialized is notable. Immigrant mothers come from societies that endorse Eastern notions of "self" that are consistent with aspects of Confucianism that essentially minimize or eliminate the role of an individual as an independent agent. Thus, they tend to emphasize sacrifice, interdependence, and conformity for the collective interest of the family and, by extension, a harmonious unity between the sexes achieved through adhering to distinct, but complementary gender roles. In contrast, their daughters have greater exposure during their formative years to the American ideals of individualism, gender equality, and self-definition. The challenge for the daughters is to redefine their mother's conception of what it means to be women to allow it to encompass the ever-broadening expectations of women in mainstream society.

ASIAN IMMIGRANT MOTHERS

Many Asian immigrant mothers who led a life of domesticity in their homelands are required to enter the work force to generate sufficient income. Their employment outside the home signifies a dramatic new role. In their homelands, women operate on a well-defined set of marital roles, in which men are expected to work, while women are to stay at home. Asia's professional system also makes it nearly impossible for women to have both a family and a career (Choi, 1994; Orenstein, 2001). However, under the new economic situation, a majority of immigrant mothers are employed outside their home (Kim & Hurh, 1998). Women's economic assimilation and entry into the work force challenge the viability of traditional gender roles and expectations as immigrant households are forced to adjust to a new family structure that is distinctly nontraditional.

Interestingly though, Asian immigrant mothers do not necessarily regard traditional gender family structure and their contribution to it as a source of subjugation and limitation (Hune, 1997; Kim & Hurh, 1998; Zhou & Nordquist, 2000). Contrary to mainstream feminist doctrines that have historically held that women's participation in the work force provides opportunity for personal self-fulfillment and emancipation from the confines of domestic duties, Asian immigrant women do not necessarily perceive their work roles as a new and autonomous activity distinct from their domestic sphere. Instead, they regard their employment to be an extension of their domestic obligations, reflecting the Asian ideal that places the success of the family, as opposed to the individual, as the paramount goal. These women also indicated that, if they had an option not to work, they would prefer to stay at home as full-time wives and mothers (Kim & Hurh, 1998), echoing the central role of motherhood in the lives of Asian women in their countries of origin (Choi, 1994).

Asian immigrant mothers recognize that their work options are limited by their lack of familiarity with the English language and American culture. Consequently, they seek employment opportunities within their ethnic communities, sometimes earning wages below minimum standard and below mean family poverty income (Zhou & Nordquist, 2000). These women further recognize that better opportunities are more appropriately suited to their children because their children will develop language facility and social familiarity through their interaction with the American education system. Their daughters, who are educated and socialized in this country, do not see the need to limit the scope of their expectations solely to their ethnic communities. Their education and socialization allow them to move toward the mainstream, and accordingly develop more mainstream expectations and seek careers for intrinsic satisfaction.

The Daughters' Assimilation Conflicts

The younger generation of women has proven to be remarkably receptive to their parental emphasis on educational and occupational advancement. Many children of immigrant parents have quickly converted their immigrant status into a professional one. Unfortunately, upward mobility of the successive generation has had painful consequences. Educational institutions have long been recognized as vehicles of acculturation. Directly and indirectly, these institutions transmit the beliefs, practices, and values that are thought to embody American ideals. Consequently, the lack of representation of ethnic and cultural values in school can foster daughters' estrangement from their parents, their roots, and their history. Additionally, the pressures to assimilate in school can force the subsequent generation to lose contact with their ethnic identity and adopt an American one. Ironically, the very stress that parents place on their children to further their citizenship process often makes the daughters strangers in both worlds by driving a wedge between their traditional values and contemporary values of American society. In order to complete the migration process, the daughters have to succeed by American standards; they have to understand and live within American society. However, this acculturation process changes the way the daughters behave within the family structure; as they become more Americanized, their mothers recognize them as being less Asian.

GENERATIONAL CONFLICTS

The younger generation's faster acculturation rate seems to cause misunderstanding and sadness. When Asian mothers are traditional and expect their daughters to keep their cultural traditions as a means of preserving their identity, pride, respect, and ties to their homelands, they are likely to experience their daughters' acculturation process with a profound sense of loss and disappointment. A number of immigrant mothers share the sentiment that they came to the United States to provide a better life for their children, and although their children clearly do have better lives, these parents feel they have lost them in the process.

Immigrant mothers' sense of losing their daughters arises out of their ambivalence about their daughters' acculturation process. Although the mothers typically desire some acculturation into the mainstream society for their children, they believe American culture is too permissive and gives the younger generation too much freedom. For example, when a daughter envisions a different life for herself, her mother is likely to view the daughter's assertion of personal choice as a selfish exercise of disobedience against her mother's parental authority and rebellion against the cultural practice of filial piety, a child's undisputed duty to observe parental authority.

Conversely, the acculturated daughters may misinterpret the significance of filial piety in Confucian societies. Zhang and Bond (1998) believed that traditional expectations within the parent-child relationship relate directly to the Confucian concept of reciprocity between family members and often are part of relationships of mutual dependence. As a result, the boundaries between Asian parents and their children are more permeable than those among American families, where there is a clear distinction between the generations (Leung, 1996). Emotional and physical separation from nuclear families tends to occur later for Asian-American families than among American families because of their less delineated distinction between the generations. This unique dyadic relationship in which the self/other boundaries are more blurred means that accomplishments, decisions, and transgressions of one family member are absorbed, shared, and reflected by every member in the family. Therefore, the collective nature of the family prevents any decision from becoming a personal choice. Every decision a daughter makes, even in personal matters such as selecting a romantic partner or a prospective career, must be weighed against her filial obligations to her parents.

Daughters' Maturation Process Intensifies Generational Conflicts

Complications arising out of the acculturated daughters' tendencies toward breaching traditional parent-child etiquette and customs expose the ubiquitous manner in which traditional rules and practices permeate the very fiber of Asian immigrant families. Young and old alike struggle with the generation gap, but the daughters often seem particularly poignant when they describe their experience because, mixed in with the daughters' differences from their mothers, is often a feeling of loss and sadness as they try to figure out how to be Asians in America. The trans-generational acculturation shift intensifies the parent-child conflicts, especially during the adolescent years when developmental stressors associated with normal adolescents striving for independence are evident.

Although all adolescents undergo identity crisis at some level, Asian-American daughters face identity conflicts while being exacerbated by the acculturation issues. The task of trying to develop their identity based on two distinct cultural perspectives, each demanding a different expectation, poses a difficult plight for the younger generation as they attempt to define who they are and how to locate themselves in mainstream society. Although identity formation is a largely unconscious process (Erikson, 1959), the daughters are painfully aware of their divided cultural loyalties. The personal question of "Who am I?" is intimately connected to how oneself identifies with and is identified by the general culture. These daughters are troubled by the thought that they might not meet others' expectations as they look beyond their families to the mainstream to define who they are. Similarly, cultural identity problems also emerge when the daughters, as young adults, begin to search for their future place in the larger society. The daughters often face conflicts in establishing themselves both as Asians and Americans, especially when immigrant success in America is measured by their ability to conform to mainstream norms. The identification issues also arise as women align themselves to political ideologies. A daughter, for example, may be proud of her Eastern heritage, but find this allegiance slipping when she begins to think about the deeply regimented, gender-based limitations endured by women in her traditional culture. Even though identity formation is a lifelong process, the search to integrate their gender and racial identity is particularly salient for children of immigrant parents because their identity synthesizes various cultural identifications.

The Paradox of Choice

Ironically, the daughters' life experience and exposure to two distinct and often conflicting cultural orientations of female gender ideals both enables and disables these women. On the one hand, they are provided opportunities to exercise vast discretion in the choices by which they define and create their identities as Asian-Americans and as women. However, this shift in cultural standards also presents these daughters with the daunting task of sifting through a multitude of options without the opportunity to avail themselves of guidance from their gender role models because their mothers have never faced the challenges required to adapt to such transgenerational and transcultural forces. For instance, the mothers can speak to the challenges of adolescence based on their own experiences, but they have no concept of what it means to be an Asian girl in an American high school. Clearly, the daughters' experience goes far beyond mere generational differences.

Daughters' Intrapsychic Conflicts

Gender identity crises stemming from generational dissonance often emerge when the daughters realize that they must differentiate themselves from their mothers' path in order to establish their own female identity. In order for the daughters to move forward, they must confront the separation guilt associated with psychically differentiating themselves from their mothers. This is a much more complicated challenge than the usual development of separation-individuation that is associated with the universal striving of a succeeding generation to differentiate itself from its parents' generation. Developmental theorists suggest that the same-sex parent is the primary influence in the formation of children's gender identity and gender-role learning. Accordingly, Asian-American daughters must separate from the very parent with whom they must identify. As a result, the daughters, while in the process of establishing their identities, often unconsciously engage in a psychic struggle in which their desire to surpass their mothers necessitates a process of disengagement which becomes psychically experienced as being equivalent to killing off their internalized representation of their mothers. The conflict between the daughter's unconscious experience of matricide-like individuation and the daughter's conscious awareness of heightened Eastern parental reverence and filial piety engenders feelings of guilt and emotional turmoil that compound the stressors already existing in the cycle of maturation.

MAINSTREAM STEREOTYPES OF ASIAN-AMERICAN WOMEN

Unfortunately, the discrepancies between the real lives of Asian-American women and popular portrayals of them in mainstream media, through works such as The Joy Luck Club, Suzy Wong, and Madame Butterfly, further contribute to the identity confusion suffered by many Asian-American women. Rather than providing real life depictions of

Asian-American women, these portrayals inundate them and the rest of contemporary America with fantastic and stereotypical images of abandonment and infanticide of Asian females, of forced prostitution or domestic servitude, and of mistreatment by Asian men and subsequent rescue by Caucasian men as characteristic of the average experiences of Asian women.

Le Espiritu (1996) asserted that such American stereotypes undermine Asian-Americans' psychological functioning and social adjustment to mainstream society. Le Espiritu opined that mainstream media have and continue to assault Asians, Americans, and Asian-Americans with fictions connoting two conflicting extremes: Asian women portrayed as demur, docile, and deferential in roles including the Geisha Girl, China Doll, and servile mail order brides; or they are portrayed as treacherous and cunning Dragon ladies, castrating martial arts sidekicks, or perpetual outsiders like those of the Yellow Peril. Le Espiritu noted that this dichotomy has permeated the sexual conceptions of Asian women, wherein they are portrayed as exotic but dainty sex objects, opium addicted prostitutes, or, as in the image of the model minorities, asexual intellectual overachievers. The pervasiveness of these images permits these stereotypes to be almost woven into the standard perception of Asian-American females, further distinguishing them from the archetype of the emancipated Caucasian-American woman.

There is no question that Asian women are embedded in perhaps the oldest, most highly developed, male-dominated kinship system in history. However, mainstream stereotypes and an oversimplified view of Asian women as merely passive, ignorant, or lacking self-esteem exemplify the denigration of women from traditional Confucian backgrounds while perpetuating distortions that parallel the phenomenon of victim blaming. Such a characterization also forecloses broader exploration of political, social, and gender stratification of Asian-American women and marginalizes their experience as a distinct group of gender and racial minority in the U.S.

QUALITATIVE DIFFERENCES IN WOMEN'S EXPERIENCES

It is important to realize that the qualitative differences in perspectives of female identity between immigrant mothers and contemporary women reflect the dynamic effects of experiences unique to each. Therefore, immigrant mothers will not have the same experiences as mainstream Caucasian women, nor will they have the same goals or opportunities. Similarly, the experiences of immigrant mothers are qualitatively different from those of their daughters'.

To begin with, immigrant mothers did not intentionally seek to enhance their status as women when they sought employment outside their home. Instead, they joined the work force out of economic necessity. In doing so, they inadvertently modified traditional gender relations and rules of engagement within the family. The mothers' views on women, however, remained fundamentally unchanged despite the structural changes to their traditional family (Chin, 2000). The experience of the daughters differs in that they have actively sought to challenge traditional patriarchal systems by enhancing their status and identity as women.

Life experiences also set immigrant mothers apart from their daughters. For immigrant mothers, issues of gender equality and inclusion are less compelling because they are preoccupied with the family's economic stability. In contrast, the daughters can exercise choices and opportunities initiated by their parents and demand inclusion and visibility in American society as Asian-American women. The daughters are in a better position to actualize America's promise of self-definition in ways that are unavailable to their immigrant mothers. Therefore, the subsequent generation generally seeks lives that are very different from those of their traditional mothers (Hune, 1997). Their intimate relationships and marriages are noted for companionship and a more egalitarian sharing of responsibilities as compared with their parents' marriages. The daughters' recognition that Confucian traditions clash with the egalitarianism and individualism they presently experience in mainstream society may cause them to reject the traditional image of a woman who gives up her own chance for self-realization, because they may believe perpetuating Confucian traditions would be counterproductive to their own achievement. Additionally, the daughters have been socialized by the mainstream to prize their individuality over conformity, self-assertion over self-sacrifice, and individual success over collective interest. Nonetheless, this trend does not mean the daughters are not ambivalent about their loyalty to their mothers and their mothers' adherence to traditional values.

As Chin (2000) aptly noted, there are many positive qualities and values inherent in traditional Confucian cultures of the immigrant mothers. While kowtowing to men may undermine their daughters' aspiration toward female empowerment, immigrant mothers' willingness to sacrifice and endure tremendous hardship to ensure that their subsequent generation has better opportunities is truly admirable. In essence, the mothers' adherence to traditional family values and maternal sacrifice has initiated a path for their daughters to see beyond the limited scope of their mothers' experience. However, by conventional standards, female strength is measured by independence and career attainment in positions once dominated by men (Talbot, 2001). Thus, the perceptions of such mothers as unwitting contributors to their own subjugation often obfuscate their desire to promote opportunities and advancements for their children. The silent strength of immigrant mothers' maternal sacrifice is often overshadowed by the overt expressions of female strength projected by mainstream images of female empowerment. Asian immigrant mothers' emphasis on maternal consciousness, along with her lack of cultural fluency and English proficiency, are hardly the image of female empowerment projected in mainstream ideology. The problem is that Asian immigrant mothers cannot stake claims in mainstream professionalism nor do they fit mainstream standards of female strength that are considered traditionally non-Asian: self-defined, independent, and powerful. Rather, they are criticized for being too maternal and not womanly enough to possess the agency and status as compared to those of contemporary women, which invariably contributes to the daughters' gender identity conflicts.

The subsequent generation's desire for the privilege that contemporary U.S. women possess in mainstream society may, in the extreme, cause a daughter to experience her mother's sacrifice as a self-negating force that draws her to choose between a restricted Asian role and a more liberated American ideal. Clearly, these daughters do not exist in a vacuum; they are exposed to the privileged status of contemporary U.S. women contrasted by fantastic portrayals of Asian-American women in contemporary media as meek, passive, and selfless. Such negative reinforcement leads some Asian-American women to reject their cultural heritage and internalized images of their mothers and ratify these self-denigrating interpretations.

The cultural divide in female images can be explained through borderline cross-cultural psychological concepts of the East and West; each as being a mutually antagonistic member of the couple unfortunately widen the cultural rifts by focusing on the extremes of each culture rather than narrowing the extensive similarities that women in each society struggle with in dealing with male privilege. Unfortunately, the daughters are also looking at their struggle as a duality when they are trying and are forced to integrate such principles that, when taken to the extreme, appear to be contradictory and mutually exclusive. Obviously, addressing this phenomenon solely from either perspective yields incomplete and imperfect explanations for the cause of the internal crises that these daughters encounter as they strive to establish themselves as a racially unique group of women. Such a limited, dualistic approach can only contribute to the ambivalence experienced by some of the daughters, who feel that they must choose between two formal contradictory characteristics of female identity, as if there were two and only two ways of defining their womanhood, instead of recognizing that their dilemma reflects the universal plight of women's struggle to be treated as equal to men, in which privileges and standards in both Confucian and contemporary American societies continue to be dominated and reinforced by models dictated by men.

RELEVANCE OF FEMINIST THERAPY IN FACILITATING A SYNTONIC GENDER IDENTITY

Feminist therapy is ideal for helping Asian-American women integrate a syntonic gender identity because it provides a conceptual framework for the social, cultural, and political forces upon the identity of women. In many ways, feminist practitioners can draw parallels within feminist history to gain insights into the Asian-American daughters' gender identity crises. As Friedan (1997) illustrated, the existential challenges that pre-feminist movement American women experienced in defining their identity began when women's sense of their individual autonomy became constrained by their roles as housewives and mothers. Women's quest for self-identity and personal autonomy led them to question who they were and what they wanted. The yearning for answers to such inquiries encouraged these women to dissect the conventional image of the American suburban housewife in order to discover the causes of their angst. This, in turn, led them to reevaluate their familial and societal relationships and the rights therewith associated, ultimately leading to a new ideological orientation whereby they began demanding rights and treatment equal to those of men, thus pioneering the forward edge of the contemporary American feminist movements.

Feminist practitioners can employ similar explorations into the sociocultural and political forces in understanding the gender identity conflicts of Asian-American women and their attempts to understand who they are as women within the context of their ethnicity as they straddle the divide between mainstream egalitarian gender values and traditional Confucian gender ideals. By highlighting the powerful role external factors play in defining women's self-identification, the therapist can help the daughters recognize that their emergent identity conflicts are fueled by a dilemma between their racial and sexual identity at a personal level and divided cultural loyalties at a societal level.

When Asian-American women present gender-identity related concerns expressed through their conflicts with their mothers, the feminist therapists can educate the daughters to understand that the distress they are feeling is due to mainstream forces present in their adopted society which are causing them to challenge many aspects of what they perceive to be their role models. In essence, feminist therapists would be facilitating the daughters to see the nexus of where societal forces affect their maturational process and intrapsychic conflicts similar to the manner in which practitioners seek to foster their patients' capacity for an observing ego. This therapeutic intervention rests on the assumption that the daughters' capacity to observe the construction and merging of their external and inner realities will raise their awareness of how external forces indelibly influence their subjective experience.

The principles of feminist therapy can serve as a catalyst to empower the daughters' gender consciousness by encouraging them to explore the historical, political, and social contexts of their mothers' and grandmothers' lives in Asia and their journey and experience in America as immigrants. Although the rise of gender consciousness in mainstream America may appeal to the daughters' sense of equality and justice, their experience as a special racial and gender minority cannot be satisfactorily bridged by ignoring the cultural and historical differences unique to each. Feminist practitioners can use their recognition of the effects of sexism and oppression on problems experienced by women to inculcate a deeper and fuller meaning into the daughters' gender and ethnic identity by encouraging them to examine the experiences of Asian-Americans' struggle with sexism and racism in the U.S., as well as the inherent sexism embedded in traditional Confucian cultures. This, in turn, will provide a context for the daughters' generational conflicts and create an impetus for their realization that they are, indeed, a new generation of women who must create precedent, rather than be guided by it.

As the daughters become more self-defining and self-determining through their realization that neither their mother's traditional female identity nor contemporary American women's experience can solely capture their experiences although they share sexual similarities with both groups of women, feminist therapists can prepare them to dissect both cultural images of female identity wherein the daughters select aspects and qualities that they deem most appropriately contribute to their establishment of their gender identity while discerning the extremes that limit their capacity to progress. The critical examination of both the contributions and limitations of each of the cultural images of female identity will provide the daughters with a new way of thinking about the explicit and implicit stratification of female ideals. Moreover, they can apply what they have learned to bridge the ambivalence and cultural chasm based on a hybrid of Eastern and Western conceptions that work synergistically. The transformative potential of Asian-American women's gender identity ultimately rests in their capacity to recognize that they are not merely trying to reconcile Western gender ideals and their Eastern heritage, but also trying to find an intellectual consensus among the vastly similar attributes that exist within two distinct cultural identities that have been defined otherwise in almost diametrically opposed principles by the extremes of their competing value systems and psychological processes. Both contemporary American and traditional Asian female images have their merits and weaknesses, but neither can comprehensively encompass all aspects of female identity and authority. This shift, from a dualistic postulation of an antithetical view of female images toward a fundamental understanding of how each cultural image reflects the universal plight of all women and women's reaction to male/female gender power differentials reinforced by male privilege, is central to the daughters' establishment of their own gender identity.

As the daughters begin to treat the various forms of female images as expressions of female identities forged in the context of social categories, sexism, and other forms of oppression, they will be able to distinguish how both Asian and American women have paradoxically attempted to arrive at a resolution to male privilege through images that are distinctly cultural; but each has employed different means in her efforts to do so: Asian women by learning to live and find power within the traditional image of motherhood and American women by demanding status and power equal to men.

CONCLUSION

In sum, Asian-American daughters' conflicts in defining their gender identity are an inevitable process for the succeeding generation as they embark on another cycle of generational transformation. The unique challenges Asian-American women face require therapists to employ multicultural feminist counseling interventions provided by feminist therapy. An integration of basic tenets of feminist therapy is vital to the daughters' development of a syntonic gender identity because it makes it possible for the daughters to identify both overt and subtle challenges and power differentials between men and women that are placed on female identity. The daughters' formation of a syntonic gender identity, in large part, depends on a fundamental understanding of male privilege in societies and the different ways women from all cultures struggle to validate their experience. The strength of feminist therapy is in its incorporation of psychological principles into feminist theory. Through their understanding of power and its interconnections among gender, race, class, and culture, feminist practitioners can help Asian-American daughters discover that the primary cause of their gender identity conflict is the damaging effects of male dominated expectations of women and each culture's masculinized view of human potential; and the secondary cause is feeling that they must choose between conflicting cultural images. The interpretative power of feminist therapy allows the subsequent generation of Asian-American women to develop new notions of womanhood by deconstructing existing cultural images and reconstructing new ones that reflect the realities of their lives as a unique racial and gender minority in the U.S.

REFERENCES

Chang, L. (1999). Gender role egalitarian attitudes in Beijing, Hong Kong, Florida and Michigan. *Journal of Cross-Cultural Psychology, 30*(6), 722-741.

Chin, J. L. (2000). *Relationships among Asian-American women.* Washington DC: American Psychological Association.

Choi, E. (1994). Status of family and motherhood for Korean women. In J. Gelb & M. L. Palley (Eds.), *Women of Japan and Korea* (pp. 189-205). Philadelphia: Temple University Press.

Erikson, E. H. (1959). *Identity and the life cycle.* New York: W. W. Norton.

Friedan, B. (1997). *The feminine mystique.* New York: W. W. Norton.

Hune, S. (1997). *Teaching Asian-American women's history.* Washington DC: American Historical Association.

Hune, S. (2000). Doing gender with a feminist gaze: Toward a historical reconstruction of Asian America. In M. Zhou & J. V. Gatewood (Eds.), *Contemporary Asian America* (pp. 413-430). New York: New York University Press.

Kim, K. C., & Hurh, W. M. (1998). The burden of double roles: Korean wives in the U.S.A. In F. Ng (Ed.), *Asian-American women and gender* (pp. 103-120). New York: Garland.

Le Espiritu, Y. (1996). *The gender lens: Asian-American women and men.* Thousand Oaks, CA: Sage.

Leung, K. (1996). The role of beliefs in Chinese culture. In M. Bond (Ed.), *The handbook of Chinese psychology* (pp. 247-262). Hong Kong: Oxford University Press.

Orenstein, P. (2001, July 1). Parasites in prêt-a-porter. *The New York Times Magazine*, 31-35.

Talbot, M. (2001, September 9). Family values: Mothers and daughters at home and at work. *The New York Times Magazine*, 54-56.

Williams, J. E., & Best, D. L. (1990). *Sex and psyche: Gender and self viewed cross-culturally*. Newbury Park, CA: Sage.

Zhang, J., & Bond, M. (1998). Personality and filial piety among college students in two Chinese societies: The added value of indigenous constructs. *Journal of Cross-Cultural Psychology, 29*(3), 402-417.

Zhou, M., & Nordquist, R. (2000). Work and its place in the lives of immigrant women: Garment workers in New York City's Chinatown. In M. Zhou & J. V. Gatewood (Eds.), *Contemporary Asian America* (pp. 254-277). New York: New York University Press.

doi:10.1300/J015v30n03_04

The Construction of South-Asian-American Womanhood: Implications for Counseling and Psychotherapy

Neesha R. Patel

SUMMARY. This article explores the ways in which South-Asian womanhood is socially constructed in the context of gendered racism in the U.S. mainstream society and gender-role expectations within the various South-Asian-American communities. These conceptions create a double bind for South-Asian-American women in which cultural loyalty and gender empowerment are placed in diametric opposition to each other. The framework of feminist multicultural counseling competence is used to discuss ways in which therapists can become more self-aware, acquire culture-specific knowledge, and develop culturally congruent interventions that incorporate the impact

Neesha R. Patel, PhD, is Assistant Professor, Counseling Department at San Francisco State University.

Address correspondence to: Neesha R. Patel, Burk Hall 524, Department of Counseling, 1600 Holloway Avenue, San Francisco State University, San Francisco, CA 94132 (E-mail: npatel@sfsu.edu).

[Haworth co-indexing entry note]: "The Construction of South-Asian-American Womanhood: Implications for Counseling and Psychotherapy." Patel, Neesha R. Co-published simultaneously in *Women & Therapy* (The Haworth Press, Inc.) Vol. 30, No. 3/4, 2007, pp. 51-61; and: *Feminist Reflections on Growth and Transformation: Asian American Women in Therapy* (ed: Debra M. Kawahara, and Oliva M. Espín) The Haworth Press, Inc., 2007, pp. 51-61. Single or multiple copies of this article are available for a fee from The Haworth Document Delivery Service [1-800-HAWORTH, 9:00 a.m. - 5:00 p.m. (EST). E-mail address: docdelivery@haworthpress.com].

Available online at http://wt.haworthpress.com

doi:10.1300/J015v30n03_05

of gendered cultural dynamics in the lives of South-Asian-American women. doi:10.1300/J015v30n03_05

KEYWORDS. South-Asian-American women, gendered racism, sexism, multicultural counseling, feminist therapy, critical consciousness

According to the U.S. Census, South-Asian Americans are now the fastest growing ethnic group within the fastest growing racial category of Asian Americans (U.S. Census, 2000). Yet, if one were to peruse the professional psychological literature, there is little guidance with regard to providing multiculturally competent services to South-Asian-American (SAA) women. The invisibility of SAA women is further perpetuated by popular notions of this group as little more than weak victims of their gender oppressive cultures (Dasgupta, 1998). The purpose of this article is to explore the gendered cultural dynamics that infuse the lives of SAA women and the consequent implications for counseling and psychotherapy. In an attempt to highlight the interplay of gender and culture, SAA women's experiences will be discussed in generalities. I would like to emphasize that these generalities are not intended to obscure the inherent variations that color the lives of SAA women. It is my hope that these thematic dynamics will be understood in the context of the individual uniqueness of each SAA woman.

WHO ARE SOUTH-ASIAN-AMERICAN WOMEN?

As a group, SAA women vary with regard to several dimensions. First, the term South Asian refers to individuals who claim their ancestry in nations as varied as Bangladesh, India, Nepal, Pakistan and Sri Lanka (Dasgupta, 1998). The regional and ethnic diversity within each of these countries further adds to the variations in cultural traditions and practices that influence the lives of SAA women. SAA women also vary with regard to their religious background and practice. Some religions that are commonly practiced among SAA women include Islam, Hinduism, Sikhism, Christianity, Buddhism, Jainism, and Zoroastrianism.

SAA women also vary with regard to their immigration histories and generational statuses. While a few SAA women immigrated to the U.S. before 1965, the majority of first generation immigrant women came to the U.S. after the racist ban against immigration from Asia was lifted by the Immigration and Naturalization Act of 1965 (Jensen, 1988). Because the U.S. immigration policies tended to prefer highly educated and skilled immigrants, the first post-1965 major wave of SAA consisted primarily of the elite, educated bourgeois of South Asia. Later, as first generation immigrants from South Asia came to the U.S. to reunite with their families or to fulfill job contracts, the socioeconomic class of the first generation SAA women began to vary. In addition to holding professional positions, more and more SAA women began to work in service positions at restaurants, ethnic grocery stores, newspaper stands, and motels.

The second generation daughters of the first generation immigrant community are becoming an increasingly larger proportion of the SAA community. These women add another layer of variation to the community of SAA women in their unique adaptation to being native to the U.S. while being raised by individuals who are not. This group of women is faced with the task of negotiating their identities and lives within the ethnic community and outside in the larger American social context. For both first and second generation SAA women, coming to terms with what it means to be "South Asian," "woman," and "American" occurs in the context of immigration histories, generational statuses, ethnic ancestry, religious beliefs, and class.

CONSTRUCTION OF SAA WOMANHOOD

Gendered Racism in the Construction of South-Asian-American Womanhood

Despite the aforementioned heterogeneity that characterizes the community of SAA women, the mainstream U.S. tends to uphold the homogeneous colonial image of SAA women as weak, passive, submissive, exotic, and subservient (Dasgupta, 1998). With regard to sexuality, SAA women are at times stereotyped as asexual and undesirable while at other times they are considered hypersexual, Kama Sutra proficient, and sexually available. Essed (1991) referred to these racist stereotypes that are gender-specific as reflective of what she termed gendered racism in the U.S.; that is, the form of racism that uniquely targets women of a particular ethnic group.

Gendered racism is not only reflected in the formation of a SAA womanhood that is objectified, but also in its relation to notions of White womanhood. According to Pyke and Johnson (2003), notions of Asian-American womanhood tend to be constructed in diametric opposition to White womanhood, where White womanhood is privileged. That is, while Asian-American women are construed as weak, passive, exotic, and submissive, White women are construed as normal, confident, self-possessed, and assertive. Given this framework, SAA women are left either to comply with an objectified stereotypical version of SA womanhood or constantly to prove that they are "not like the others" and risk being perceived as "acting White."

Transnational Constitutions of Gendered South-Asian Traditions

The construction of SAA womanhood is further complicated by the first generation South-Asian-American community's tendency to essentialize and homogenize the respective South Asian cultures (Dasgupta, 1998). This tendency is reflected in comments that are commonly made by members of the SA communities such as, "You're becoming too American," or "You are being so Indian." These comments demonstrate the development of a SA culture that is created in dynamic relationship to and in contrast with the SA community's perceptions of a hegemonic "American" mainstream culture. As the appointed bearers of culture, and more specifically, as the "face" of the community, SAA women are particularly affected by these cultural constructions (Dasgupta, 1998; Kallivayalil, 2004). Oftentimes, SAA women are expected to adhere to and transmit those aspects of SA "tradition" that are designed to control their sexuality and behavior. For example, compared to SAA sons, SAA daughters are subject to greater restrictions on their sexual and social behavior and are expected to be more obedient and attentive to their family's needs (Dasgupta, 1998; Ayyub, 2000).

According to Espin (1999), essentialized "traditions" that are deployed in a gendered manner may be a product of the immigrant community's attempts to cope with the chaotic transition of immigration into a racist mainstream U.S. society. For SAA, considering the legacy of immigration history in which only the highly skilled and educated "model minority" were permitted to enter the U.S. in order to "work hard" and meet the needs of corporate America, control of SAA women's behavior may be an attempt to create a flawless and homogeneous image of SA culture to safeguard the community's standing in the racially stratified U.S. society. Additionally, in a societal context in which SAA men are perceived as racially inferior and emasculated, controlling women's behavior may also serve as a way to assert sexist notions of masculine power. Furthermore, the backdrop of the immense loss that is inherent in the process of immigration may also contribute to the SAA community's impulse to preserve tradition by tightening restrictions on women's behavior as they face the threat of losing even more in a dominant cultural context that pulls for homogenization (Dasgupta, 1998).

The Issue of Cultural Sensitivity vs. Gender Empowerment

The dichotomy between cultural loyalty and personal liberation for SAA women is further exacerbated by what Espin (1999) refers to as the third oppression. The third oppression involves the dismissal of gender oppression in the name of cultural sensitivity. This type of oppression is evidenced in U.S. court cases in which the "cultural defense" is used to acquit Asian-American men who engage in violence against Asian-American women by labeling that violence as a cultural practice (Leti, 1996). Consequently, many SAA women live with the threat that the U.S. courts will tolerate violence committed against them if it is committed by a man from their ethnic community.

Such "cultural sensitivity" conceives of SA culture as inherently sexist and therefore inferior to U.S. mainstream culture and stems from the denial of two important facts. First, sexism is just as much a part of the mainstream U.S. culture as it is of mainstream SA culture. For example, the U.S. media tends to selectively attend to sexist practices such as honor killings and female infanticide in South Asia, while denying the fact that one in three women who are murdered in the U.S. are murdered by their male intimate partners and the fact that the Equal Rights Amendment that guarantees the equal treatment of men and women under the law is still not a part of the U.S. Constitution (U.S. Department of Health and Human Services, 2003; Kaminer, 2001). The second fact is that women's empowerment is just as much a part of South Asian histories and cultures as it is a part of U.S. history and culture. For example, while women's suffrage is often touted as a sign of the ascendancy of U.S. culture, South Asian countries have had several female prime ministers lead their nations compared to the U.S. which has yet to elect even one female president.

Implications for SAA Women

The aforementioned sociocultural forces result in the denial of those aspects of South Asian (SA) culture that are empowering of women while promoting a concept of SAA womanhood that assumes that SA culture is inferior, inherently sexist and restricting of women's behavior. When internalized, this notion of SA womanhood that obscures any variation in either SAA womanhood or White American womanhood can result in a psychological double bind for SAA women. That is, given that SAA women will never be accepted as American (read: White), they may begin to view themselves as passive, exotic, submissive, and either hypersexual or asexual. Alternatively, they may feel like a failure because they are unable to live up to this unrealistic caricature. Furthermore, perceptions of SAA women as sexually available, subservient, and submissive can leave them vulnerable to sexual violence, exploitation, and mistreatment (Jones & Shorter-Gooden, 2003).

Interpersonal interactions rooted in gendered racism have been shown to have deleterious effects on SAA women's psychological health. For instance, Iyer and Haslam (2003) have found that racial teasing can predict body image dissatisfaction among SAA women. Additionally, race-based sexual harassment among Asian-American women has been linked to feelings of shame, worthlessness, distrust, and guilt (Chan, 1987).

SAA women who resist the objectifying notion of SA womanhood may be perceived as denying their ethnic heritage or "acting White," and "not like the others." Due to the internalization of the dichotomy between SA culture and gender empowerment, SAA women who behave in gender empowering ways may feel isolated from their ethnic community and fellow SAA women. For second-generation women, a primary link to one's ethnicity is one's family, and resistance to restricting conceptions of SA womanhood may mean painful disconnection from family members (Dasgupta, 1998). Additionally, they may be left with a sense of having to constantly prove that they are indeed different, and therefore, "better" than their SAA sisters.

Both compliance with and resistance to the stereotypes of SAA women are rooted in an internalization of the racist and sexist notion of SAA womanhood. Maintaining this idea of SAA womanhood can result in the fragmentation of SAA women's ethnic and gender aspects of themselves. Additionally, this internalization denies SAA women their sense of agency in defining themselves.

IMPLICATIONS FOR COUNSELING AND PSYCHOTHERAPY

For SAA women, notions of SA womanhood are deeply embedded in common presenting concerns such as body image satisfaction, relationships, sexuality, and career exploration. In order to work through such issues, SAA women may need to engage in the process of shifting from an objective definition of themselves to a subjective definition of themselves. From a multicultural feminist perspective, psychotherapy can facilitate an individual's efforts to empower themselves through such redefinitions. The following is a discussion of how feminist therapists can use the three prongs of multicultural competence (exploration of one's biases, obtaining culturally-specific knowledge and utilizing culturally congruent interventions) to create an empowering, growing, and healing therapeutic context in their work with SAA women.

Therapist, Know Thyself

The foundational step in becoming a multiculturally competent therapist is becoming aware of one's own biases and assumptions (Sue, Arredondo, & McDavis, 1992). In an effort to develop an egalitarian relationship with our clients, we must be willing to acknowledge that both client and therapist are infused with racist and sexist ideology that positions SAA women as inferior compared to White women. We must examine the ways in which both sexism and racism have served to construct our notion of SA womanhood–particularly as it relates to our own racial/gender identity. We must ask ourselves whether our racial/gender status is privileged or oppressed in the U.S. and what that might mean about how we construe notions of womanhood in our own cultural groups. Given the power differential between client and therapist and the fact that the therapeutic dyad is a microcosm of the larger social context, we need to recognize that colluding with racist and sexist notions of SA womanhood can harm our clients. Such collusions can result in reinforcing psychologically damaging notions of SAA womanhood and recreating oppressive conditions in the therapeutic context.

Women's Empowerment in South-Asian Cultural Context

The second aspect of multicultural competence involves therapists taking the responsibility to gain culturally-specific knowledge regarding their clients. In working with SAA women, we, as therapists, need to go beyond looking to our clients to teach us about an essentialized concept of SA womanhood, to ask ourselves what we know about the sociocultural influences that can shape stereotypical notions of SA womanhood in the U.S.

Additionally, we need to ask ourselves if we are aware of SA women who are empowered within a South-Asian historical and cultural context. If not, we must learn of the myriad of images and symbols of women's empowerment that are embedded in a South-Asian context. For example, Dasgupta (1998) described the concept of the "virangana." The virangana refers to the concept of the brave warrior woman and is reflected in images of Hindu goddesses such as Durga and Kali, Muslim female freedom fighters in colonial times such as Halima Khatun and Badrunnesssa Begum, and more contemporary women such as the courageous writer Taslima Nasrin of Bangladesh, global activist Vandana Shiva of India, and the first woman in the world to become prime minister of a nation, Sirimavo Bandaranaike of Sri Lanka (Dasgupta, 1998).

Beyond South Asia, SAA women in the U.S. are also using South Asian cultural symbols as tools for empowerment. For example, Chaudhary (1998) described a second generation Pakistani American Muslim woman she interviewed who chooses to wear a hijab (a veil) contrary to her family's wishes. The hijab is often considered a symbol of the oppression of women in the eyes of the West. However, for this woman, the hijab is a tool to defend against the sexual objectification she experiences from the mainstream. Additionally, she uses the hijab to gain voice and empowerment in her campus Muslim student organization by demonstrating her identification with Islam. Indeed, in this climate of anti-Islamic hostility, to fail to recognize the courage and bravery inherent in the choice to wear the hijab is a blatant disregard for the ways in which SAA women are demonstrating courage and strength in their lives.

Tools for Building Critical Consciousness

The third prong of multicultural competence involves the use of culturally congruent interventions in providing mental health services to SAA women. As we use various feminist techniques to help SAA women build critical consciousness, it is imperative that we, as therapists, be cognizant of the sociopolitical context in which we conduct these interventions.

From a feminist therapeutic perspective, the uses of gender-role analysis and power analysis are techniques that are used to help clients build critical consciousness (Worrell & Remer, 1992). These techniques are aimed at uncovering the sexism that adversely affects various aspects of women's lives. In using these tools with SAA women, we must be careful not to limit such an analysis to the realm of the SAA family and ethnic community. A limited focus in this regard may inadvertently reinforce the racist notion that SA culture is inherently sexist in contrast to mainstream U.S. culture which is presumed to be free of sexism and therefore superior to SA culture. Hence, an examination of the role of sexism in SAA women's lives must also incorporate an analysis of the sexism and gendered racism that is inherent in U.S. society that also affects SAA women's lives.

As therapists, we must also be aware of the impact of the use of the words "feminism" or "feminist" in working with SAA women. According to Mohanty (1991), the term "feminism" is closely tied to western notions of womanhood for some SAA women. As such, when asked to explore "feminist" conceptions of womanhood in a SA context, some SAA women may perceive this as an exploration of the ways in which western notions of womanhood are played out in SA cultures. In order to elicit more culturally-embedded symbols, words such as "strong woman," "brave woman," "adventurous woman," and "equality" may be more culturally meaningful for some SAA women. Additionally, SAA women may conceive of strength in a more collectivistic framework in which interdependence is seen as requiring more strength than independence. For example, a SAA woman who chooses to forgo a promotion at work to take care of her ailing mother may perceive herself as stronger than if she had chosen the self-promoting option of career advancement over the collective responsibility of caring for family members.

Finally, another intervention that may serve to foster growth and development of an empowering sense of SA womanhood is exposing SAA women to information and experiences in which SAA women act as empowered agents of change. For example, exposure to profiles of SAA women leaders such as Shamita Das Dasgupta, who is one of the cofounders of Manavi–the first organization in the U.S. to address the issue of violence against South-Asian-American women, or Urvashi Vaid, who was the leader of the National Gay and Lesbian Task Force, may provide a model of gender empowerment that is inherently SAA. With regard to activities, SAA women who are exposed to opportunities to work in SAA-based organizations geared towards women's empowerment also report a shift from viewing themselves as passive recipients of cultural "traditions" to active agents of women's empowerment in a

South-Asian-American context (Rudrappa, 2004). Such information and experiences that integrate SA cultural heritage, personal liberation and gender empowerment may be particularly helpful to SAA women as they work toward integrating their ethnic and gender identities.

CONCLUSION

In conclusion, I would like to quote bell hooks (1990):

> The process of becoming subjects [as opposed to objects] emerges as one comes to understand how structures of domination work in one's own life, as one develops critical thinking and critical consciousness, as one invents new, alternative habits of being and resists from that marginal space of difference inwardly defined.

In this quote, bell hooks speaks to the process of building critical consciousness as a means by which one can begin to free oneself from the shackles of what Wade Nobles (1985) called conceptual incarceration–the unwitting adoption of erroneous views, concepts, and theories about one's culture, the dominant culture, and the world. The techniques of feminist multicultural counseling provide a useful framework to guide therapists to help SAA women develop with this process. It is hoped that these techniques, guided by an understanding of the gendered cultural dynamics that infuse the lives of SAA women, will allow for the creation of a therapeutic space that is truly emancipatory and healing for SAA women.

REFERENCES

Ayyub, R. (2000). Domestic violence in the South Asian Muslim immigrant population in the United States. *Journal of Social Distress and the Homeless, 9*(3), 237-248.

Chan, C. S. (1987). Asian American women: Psychological responses to sexual exploitation and cultural stereotypes. *Women & Therapy, 6*(4), 33-38.

Chaudhary, L. (1998). "We are graceful swans who can also be crows": Hybrid identities of Pakistani Muslim women. In S. D. Dasgupta (Ed.), *A patchwork shawl: Chronicles of South Asian women in America* (pp. 46-61). New Brunswick, NJ: Rutgers University Press.

Dasgupta, S. D. (1998). *A patchwork shawl: Chronicles of South Asian women in America.* New Brunswick, NJ: Rutgers University Press.

Espín, O. M. (1999). *Women crossing boundaries: A psychology of immigration and the transformations of sexuality.* New York: Routledge.

Essed, P. (1991). *Understanding everyday racism.* Newbury Park, CA: Sage.

hooks, b. (1990). *Yearning: Race, gender, and cultural politics.* Boston: South End Press.

Iyer, D. S., & Haslam, N. (2003). Body image and eating disturbance among South Asian-American women: The role of racial teasing, *International Journal of Eating Disorders, 34*(1), 142-147.

Jensen, L. (1988). Patterns of immigration and public assistance utilization, 1970-1980. *International Migration Review, 22*(1), 51-83.

Jones, C., & Shorter-Gooden, K. (2003). *Shifting: The double lives of black women in America.* New York: HarperCollins.

Kallivayalil, D. (2004). Gender and cultural socialization in Indian immigrant families in the United States. *Feminism and Psychology, 14*(4), 535-559.

Kaminer, W. (2001). Equal rights postponement. *The American Prospect, 12*(6). Retrieved January 9, 2005, from http://www.prospect.org/print-friendly/print/V12/16/kaminer-w.html

Leti, V. (1996). Talking 'culture': Gender, race, nation, and the politics of multiculturalism. *Columbia Law Review, 96*(6), 1572-1618.

Mohanty, C. (1991). Under western eyes: Feminist scholarship and colonial discourses. In C. Mohanty, A. Russo, & L. Torres (Eds.), *Third world women and the politics of feminism* (pp. 51-80). Bloomington, IN: Indiana University Press.

Nobles, W. W. (1985). *Africanity and the black family: The development of a theoretical model.* Oakland, CA: The Institute for the Advanced Study of Black Family Life and Culture.

Pyke, K. D., & Johnson, D. L. (2003). Asian American women and racialized femininities: "Doing" gender across cultural worlds. *Gender and Society, 1*(1), 33-53.

Rudrappa, S. (2004). Radical caring in an ethnic shelter: South Asian American women workers at Apna Ghar, Chicago. *Gender and Society, 18*(5), 588-609.

Sue, D. W., Arredondo, P., & McDavis, R. J. (1992). Multicultural competencies and standards: A call to the profession. *Journal of Multicultural Counseling and Development, 20,* 64-88.

U.S. Census Bureau (2000). *Statistical Abstract of the United States: 2000* (120th ed.). Washington, DC: U.S. Government Printing Office.

U.S. Department of Health and Human Services (2003). *Costs of intimate partner violence against women in the United States.* Atlanta, GA: Author. Retrieved January 9, 2005, from http://www.cdc.gov/ncipc/pub-res/ipv_cost/ipv.htm

Worrell, J., & Remer, P. (1992). *Perspectives in therapy: An empowerment model for women.* Chichester, England: Wiley.

doi:10.1300/J015v30n03_05

Psychotherapy with Filipinas

Patricia Heras

SUMMARY. This article focuses on therapeutic work with second-generation Filipino women (Filipinas). These clients are particularly vulnerable to errors resulting from the therapist's lack of cultural competence. These clients present to their therapists as having acculturated to the mainstream culture, which may contribute to the clinicians' assumptions of assimilation. When the roles of ethnicity, culture, and oppression are minimized, errors in therapeutic assessment may occur. Important areas to consider when working with Filipinas include family matters, gender roles, intergenerational conflict, acculturation, and ethnic identity. A composite case example illustrates these areas in a therapeutic relationship. Recommendations for therapeutic practice with similar clients are included. doi:10.1300/J015v30n03_06 *[Article copies available for a fee from The Haworth Document Delivery Service: 1-800-HAWORTH. E-mail address: <docdelivery@haworthpress.com> Website: <http://www.HaworthPress.com> © 2007 by The Haworth Press, Inc. All rights reserved.]*

KEYWORDS. Filipino American women, Filipinas, psychotherapy, multicultural counseling, treatment

---

Patricia Heras, PhD, is a psychologist in private practice in San Diego, CA.

Address correspondence to: Patricia Heras, PhD, 5665 Oberlin Drive, Suite 201, San Diego, CA 92121 USA (E-mail: pherasphd@aol.com).

[Haworth co-indexing entry note]: "Psychotherapy with Filipinas." Heras, Patricia. Co-published simultaneously in *Women & Therapy* (The Haworth Press, Inc.) Vol. 30, No. 3/4, 2007, pp. 63-73; and: *Feminist Reflections on Growth and Transformation: Asian American Women in Therapy* (ed: Debra M. Kawahara, and Oliva M. Espín) The Haworth Press, Inc., 2007, pp. 63-73. Single or multiple copies of this article are available for a fee from The Haworth Document Delivery Service [1-800-HAWORTH, 9:00 a.m. - 5:00 p.m. (EST). E-mail address: docdelivery@haworthpress.com].

Available online at http://wt.haworthpress.com

doi:10.1300/J015v30n03_06

INTRODUCTION

This article focuses on Filipino American women (Filipinas) who were born in the United States of Filipino-born immigrant parents. These second-generation clients are particularly vulnerable to errors resulting from the therapist's inaccurate assessment of the role of culture in the clients' lives. Often, cultural differences between Filipinas and mainstream U.S. culture are overlooked or minimized because the language barrier is not present. While therapists generally understand the importance of cultural competence, particularly when working with immigrant populations, these second-generation clients may present to their therapists as acculturated to the mainstream culture, which can contribute to the clinicians' assumptions of assimilation. Working therapeutically with non-immigrant ethnic populations can be more challenging, as the role of culture in shaping the personality and behavior of the clients is less evident. When the roles of ethnicity, culture, and oppression are minimized, errors in therapeutic assessment may occur.

Filipina psychotherapy clients are sorting through their bicultural identities. They are clarifying how to deal more effectively with the world given their familial cultural values. Filipinas coming to therapy are often beleaguered with interpersonal issues that raise questions on the boundary between self and others. Often, they are reconciling harsh childhood histories with numerous episodes of parental assistance and support. Many of the clients report adolescent experiences of cruel verbal criticism or excessive physical discipline, yet their parents may have purchased new cars for them at 16, paid for college, and provided child care when needed.

My clinical approach is to help the Filipina filter her past through a cultural lens to understand her present, thereby empowering the choices she has made and will make. Crucial areas to consider when working with second-generation Filipinas include gender roles, family matters, intergenerational conflict, and ethnic identity.

Gender Roles

Filipinas share cultural similarities with other Asian groups, such as the importance of the family, loyalty to and interdependence with the family, patterns of communication, and the primacy of interpersonal harmony. However, unlike other countries in Asia, the Philippines was not dominated by Confucian philosophy or Buddhism. Family structure in the Philippines incorporates a bilateral kinship system;

thus, lineage comes from both the mother and the father. These factors increase the value of women and the importance of their role in society. At the same time, religion (predominantly Catholic and Muslim) has inhibited and controlled the sexual and social behavior of women. Thus, while education and economic participation are encouraged for Filipinas, social and interpersonal behavior is strictly restricted and proscribed. If a Filipina is to be a "good girl," then she must remain sexually chaste until marriage, and get along and maintain harmony with others.

For Filipinas, gender roles become more defined during adolescence. Adolescent Filipino boys are allowed to date earlier, stay out longer, and are under less supervision than their female counterparts. Women are expected to remain closely involved with their families, and are generally subject to close supervision in their social interactions. For example, in one case, the parents of a Filipina client insisted that she refuse a scholarship to an Ivy League university because of the geographic distance from home. In another case, the parents purchased an apartment for their daughter just after college graduation, but visited her apartment daily. On the one hand, Filipinas are encouraged to achieve academically, economically, and pursue career goals. At the same time, they are expected to remain close (geographically and emotionally) to the family, leading at times to difficult personal and professional choices.

Family Matters

For Filipinas, the initial group with which they identify and the one which remains central throughout their life is the family. Filipinas derive a great deal of security from family bonds not only emotionally, but economically and socially. Poor economic conditions have reinforced loyalty to and dependency on the family and kin group (Almirol, 1982). Despite their high levels of educational attainment, Filipinas have more difficulty finding jobs commensurate with their education, training, and experience than do White Americans (Bradshaw, 1994). Economic necessity coupled with experiences of racism force Filipinas to depend on the family to protect them from the traumas inherent in the cultural adaptation process, and to provide social status, honor, and a sense of belonging. The therapist may thus observe a circular process in which existing values of dependency and reliance on the family are further intensified by experiences of discrimination.

Intergenerational Conflict, Acculturation, and Ethnic Identity

Family conflict created by the cultural differences between immigrant parents and their American-born children is a substantial factor in the mental health of Filipinas. Although these clients are not dealing with the cultural adjustments and transitions that their immigrant parents had to face, they have to navigate and incorporate conflicting familial and societal pressures. A government survey indicated that in San Diego, Filipina teenagers had the highest rate of contemplating, planning, and attempting suicide when compared to all other ethnic groups (Center for Disease Control, 1993, 1995, 1997, 1999). The available literature suggests that intergenerational cultural differences in acculturation contribute to family dysfunction, which then may also contribute to suicidal behaviors of Filipina youth (Espiritu, 1994; Heras & Revilla, 1994; Rumbaut, 1995; Wolfe, 1997). These studies also reported high rates of depression and low self-esteem scores for Filipina American second-generation youth.

Several factors influence the increasing psychological stress experienced by Filipinas. First, both adolescent and young-adult Filipinas have to arbitrate between incompatible and antagonistic demands of the dominant and Filipino cultures. In the White American culture, independence, direct expression of conflict, and individualism are encouraged. In contrast, Filipino culture emphasizes family closeness, conformation to family norms, and avoidance of the direct expression of conflict. Therefore, Filipina teenagers expressing discontent with family rules may be seen as rebellious and disrespectful. Their preference to socialize with peers or choose a college out of their local area may be seen as a rejection of the family. Consequently, a Filipina raised to be dependent on the family, yet exposed to the importance of independent thinking and behavior by the dominant American culture, will experience a considerable amount of internal tension. Her parents' inability to understand and validate the child's conflicts and depression, coupled with the preference for keeping problems within the family, limit the young Filipina's options for problem resolution.

Secondly, it has been suggested that by the second generation, group identification has weakened (Sue & Sue, 1988). Unlike the first generation, there is little memory of or familiarity with one's country of origin. For example, most second-generation Filipinas have little firsthand knowledge of or about the Philippines. They generally do not speak Tagalog or any of the other Filipino dialects (Strobel, 1995). Filipino immigrants, in their desire to assimilate, usually speak to their children in English. Thus, the children become monolingual in English, at best understanding only a few Filipino phrases. This language deficit serves to further weaken ethnic identity (Revilla, 1995) and to distance Filipinas from their cultural heritage. Increasing role or value conflicts, without the security of firm group identification, contribute to the ethnic identity issues observed in Filipinas.

Ethnic identity is a dynamic process of intrapsychic and interpersonal relatedness to multiple social systems, which include the family, one's ethnic group, other ethnic groups, and larger social and political institutions. Second-generation Filipinas are engaged in actively and continually integrating family cultural values with that of the mainstream culture. For Filipino Americans as a visible minority, having a sense of ethnic belonging is crucial "to prevent social alienation and self estrangement" (Sodowsky, Kwan, & Pannu, 1995, p. 137). Yet, this necessary and ongoing task of ethnocultural identification is complicated by the Philippines' long history of Spanish and American colonization (Rimonte, 1997; Root, 1997). This lengthy history, which extends over 450 years, left a legacy of internalized oppression which is further exacerbated for Filipino Americans by experiences of racism (Strobel, 1997). The result of this history of colonization is an uneasy and insecure sense of ethnic identity that continues to beleaguer Filipino Americans today (Revilla, 1997). Most Filipino immigrants have minimal education on the Philippines' history and culture, and thus are unable to teach their American-born children the historical knowledge that is vital to cultural identity. This weak national-identity aspect of the pre-migration experience of Filipino immigrants, coupled with immigrant parents choosing to speak to their children in English, further weakens ethnic affiliation (Min, 1999).

This fragile ethnic identity leads a Filipina to depend even more on her family for a sense of belonging and safety both personally and socially. Thus, intergenerational conflict is experienced by Filipinos as particularly destructive for the family. Dependency and family closeness, while supportive, can also lead to a restrictive development of the self. The following composite case illustrates these gender, family, and ethnic identity issues.

CASE STUDY

Thelma (a pseudonym) is a 32-year-old Filipina initially referred by her physician after she overdosed on medication. She took the medication to "rest" and avoid dealing with problems at home and at work. Thelma has been married for 12 years, has three children, and works as a hospital manager.

Thelma was deeply ashamed of having overdosed on medication; she did not like to call it a suicide attempt. She believed her overdose demonstrated that she was weak and lacking in self-control. At intake, she complained of irritability, fatigue, and lethargy. She was easily bothered by her children. She was the youngest of three children and raised as a strict Catholic. Her parents emigrated from the Philippines in 1960; her father was in the military and her mother worked as a clerk. Thelma described her father as aggressive and highly critical, but not physically violent. He was the family disciplinarian, conservative and traditional in his beliefs. She described her mother as passive and over-protective.

Thelma described her years in junior high and high school as troubled. She felt unattractive and her parents were very strict with her. Physical and verbal affection were seldom displayed. She was often criticized for being "loose," meaning promiscuous. She often lied about her whereabouts and activities to her parents. She had one serious relationship in high school that ended with her boyfriend's betrayal; she attributed this rejection as confirmation of her unattractiveness. She had an unwanted pregnancy while in college, but an abortion was not an option. Her parents were very angry about the pregnancy and planned to send her out of the city to avoid embarrassment with the neighbors. This response from her parents hurt her deeply. She and her then boyfriend (now husband) married.

She was able to complete college with her family's support. Her mother cared for her child, and her parents rented the couple a home. She felt grateful for her parents' support, and guilty about her desire for greater independence from them. It was her parents' decision where she lived, and they also gave advice about homes, loans, and vacations. She generally complied with their recommendations. Her extended-family members visited her almost every weekend. She found it difficult to ask them for help (with cooking, cleaning, or buying groceries).

Despite her management position at work, Thelma felt disregarded by the management team. When the company she worked for went through a reorganization, her position was not included in the executive team, making her feel like a failure. She knew that at work she preferred to avoid conflict, and that her passive style did not engender confidence in the quality of her work.

DISCUSSION

Initial Focus

As the first visit is crucial when working with Asian clients (Sue & Sue, 1988), the therapeutic stance I adopt with my clients is to be personable and respectful. The emphasis is on joining and developing the relationship. The literature suggests that Filipino clients respond favorably to therapists' expression of personal warmth (Tompar-Tiu & Sustento-Seneriches, 1995). I answer questions about my educational and cultural background that may be seen as intrusive by other therapists. Confidentiality is explained thoroughly. This is particularly important when one is from the same ethnic group and there is uneasiness about social interactions in the community. (As a Filipina psychologist, I am aware of the tension that can occur when I meet Filipina clients unexpectedly at community functions.) It is critical to address any immediate dilemmas and end the first session by providing hope.

In the first visit, Thelma spoke slowly and quietly. She often paused and seemed to be observing my non-verbal reactions. I did not ask about the suicide attempt (although her suicidality was assessed) and instead focused on her concerns and treatment goals.

Cultural and Family Dynamics

In the subsequent sessions, she talked about her parents and upbringing guardedly, making remarks such as "I don't want to sound like I am blaming them," and "I feel terrible talking about them this way." Feelings of betraying the family by discussing family secrets are common among Filipinas. Feelings of disloyalty may surface as clients talk about experiences of harsh parenting. Pacing questions and keeping them to a level that clients can tolerate are important in the early phase of treatment.

At the onset of therapy, Thelma discussed her upbringing and family values, and we compared her experience with that of the dominant culture. This psycho-educational approach in the early phase of treatment allowed for future conversations about normative differences between her individual and family system and that of the mainstream U.S. culture. It also increased her confidence as she began a process of defining and framing problems from a multicultural, feminist perspective that reflected her experience. This perspective provided fluidity in our conversations about her objective and subjective realities, and enabled her to make thoughtful choices on values and behavior.

Therapeutic Themes

Thelma realized that she had married to avoid the shame of being an unwed mother. She was naïve about her body, sex, and sexuality. She was conflicted about how to raise her daughter without repressing her sexuality. Clarifying her own cultural beliefs on sexuality in a manner that supported Thelma's emerging identity was an important goal of treatment.

A major theme in her therapy involved clarifying the boundaries between her individual needs and those of the collective. Making decisions to honor her increasing self-awareness when group demands were present was an ongoing struggle for her. She often felt unsure of her decisions. She had a strong need to have a clear boundary between herself and others. To Thelma this meant setting clear limits with others and herself, such as not tolerating unpleasant or offensive behavior, or over-performing to please others. She was eager to know how to simultaneously take care of herself and others. She asked me, as her therapist, to set limits for her, preferring to avoid the ambiguity of struggling with this necessary developmental process for Filipinas. Clarifying and determining where and when to set limits between individual needs and collective demands is an important part of self-definition and identity. This process was further complicated by her difficulty expressing conflict. Like other Filipinas who are raised in authoritarian families, she experienced marked discomfort and anxiety verbalizing her thoughts and feelings when they contradicted or challenged others, particularly authority figures. Thelma experienced anxiety before disagreeing with her father's or boss' opinion. She had been raised not to question or challenge male authority figures. Empowering her to test new behaviors that expanded her definition of culturally congruent expressions of anger expanded her behavioral repertoire.

Outcome

Thelma completed therapy after nine months; subsequently she has come in occasionally for brief, issue-related visits. She was cleared of her depression and more clearly able to articulate her thoughts and feelings on a broad range of issues. Her identity as a Filipina was strengthened with her increased understanding of her family's culture. She was more confident and assertive about her values and opinions. Her self-doubt was replaced with positive acceptance of her reservations as unique to her processing style. Although it was still difficult for her to challenge her parents, she felt more peaceful when she chose not to dispute them. She was verbalizing her sexual needs with her husband, and aware that she needed to allow her daughters to ask her questions about their emerging sexuality.

In the course of treatment, Thelma developed the capacity to observe her own reactions to situations and interpersonal interactions. This increased self-awareness allowed her to experiment with new behaviors. This skill occurred only after the therapeutic relationship was sufficiently developed. Her ability to reject and challenge some of my suggestions was reinforced. These behaviors–challenging my authority, identifying personal behavioral goals, choosing what conflicts she engaged in–were in alignment with the treatment goal of helping her to develop a viable bicultural self and empowering her to make and accept culturally relevant choices.

POINTS TO CONSIDER WHEN WORKING WITH SECOND-GENERATION FILIPINA AMERICANS

This composite case study illustrates a number of key issues for consideration in therapeutic practice with second-generation Filipinas, particularly along the major themes of family matters, gender roles, intergenerational conflict, acculturation, and ethnic identity:

- Conflict around self-definition and boundaries is to be expected given the primacy of family closeness and dependency. Overall, second-generation Filipinas may find that continued deference to first-generation family is appropriate, respectful, and/or easiest. At the same time, developing a bicultural self-definition and boundary determination is vital for mental health.
- Second-generation Filipinas generally experience intergenerational conflict. It is essential that this process be normalized as part of the acculturation process.
- Conflicting expectations are also likely around gender roles, academic and career distinctions, control of sexuality by the family, and the pressure to remain close to home. Realization of the normalcy of these conflicts, and development of an ability to navigate

such conflicts differentially depending upon the setting, will assist in these Filipinas' development.

- Filipinas are often unfamiliar with verbally expressing conflict. This, coupled with their familiarity with authoritarian structures, contributes to a style that presents as compliant. Mediation between the two is a likely outcome, in which deference to family may continue, while development of an ability to verbalize conflict in other life situations will likely assist in acculturation if the client chooses to do so.
- Development of an ability to selectively reframe behaviors that may be seen as culturally appropriate for Filipinos, but dysfunctional in American culture, such as passivity (valuing harmony) and dependency (family closeness), is useful. Because selective rather than unilateral adaptation is most helpful to minimize intergenerational and intercultural conflict, the development of an understanding and awareness of such conflictual situations and the choices available for selective behavioral adaptation are key to a more sophisticated, situational approach to such issues.
- Filipina clients are empowered when they understand the reasons for their behavior and their multicultural and intergenerational choices. Thus, conscious awareness and active choice-making are preferable to simply redirecting behaviors and choices unilaterally.

The therapist assists the Filipina client to actively and consciously make choices that shape behavior and relationships. Ideally, the Filipina client in therapy develops the skill and discernment to make such choices situationally, particularly in light of the intercultural and intergenerational issues involved in each relationship. Choice leads to increased self-definition and empowerment. Increased self-definition and empowerment inform and avail further options and choices.

Through this process, the Filipina develops greater and fuller awareness of how she can become and be herself, exercising a range of options to honor cultural and generational traditions where appropriate, while developing a broader, multicultural self with this wider range of options at her disposal.

Finally, the therapist needs to pay attention to his or her own intergenerational, gendered, and intercultural biases and definitions of health. This self-awareness, equally helpful to the therapist, ensures that the client is not further conflicted by the unconscious assertion of additional intergenerational, gendered, and/or intercultural biases with which she is already attempting to cope.

REFERENCES

Almirol, E. (1982). Rights and obligations in Filipino American families. *Journal of Comparative Family Studies, 8*, 291-306.

Bradshaw, C. (1994). Asian and Asian American women: Historical and political considerations in psychotherapy. In L. Comas-Diaz & B. Greene (Eds.), *Women of color: Integrating ethnic and gender identities in psychotherapy* (pp. 72-113). New York: Guilford Press.

Center for Disease Control (1993). *Youth at risk behavior survey.* San Diego: San Diego City Schools. Retrieved February, 1994, from http://www.cdc.gov/yrbss

Center for Disease Control (1995). *Youth at risk behavior survey.* San Diego: San Diego City Schools. Retrieved February, 1996, from http://www.cdc.gov/yrbss

Center for Disease Control (1997). *Youth at risk behavior survey.* San Diego: San Diego City Schools. Retrieved February, 1998, from http://www.cdc.gov/yrbss

Center for Disease Control (1999). *Youth at risk behavior survey.* San Diego: San Diego City Schools. Retrieved February, 2000, from http://www.cdc.gov/yrbss

Espiritu, Y. L. (1994). The intersection of race, ethnicity, and class: The multiple identities of second generation Filipino Americans. *Identities, 1*, 249-273.

Heras, P., & Revilla, L. (1994). Acculturation, generational status, and family environment of Filipino-Americans: A study on cultural adaptation. *Family Therapy, 21*, 130-138.

Min, P. G. M. (1999). Ethnicity: Concepts, theories, and trends. In P. G. M. Min & R. Kim (Eds.), *Struggle for ethnic identity: Narratives by Asian American professionals* (pp. 16-46). Walnut Creek, CA: Alta Mira Press.

Revilla, L. (1997). Filipino American identity: Transcending the crisis. In M. P. P. Root (Ed.), *Filipino Americans: Transformation and identity* (pp. 95-111). Thousand Oaks, CA: Sage.

Rimonte, N. (1997). Colonialism's legacy: The inferiorizing of the Filipino. In M.P P. Root (Ed.), *Filipino Americans: Transformation and identity* (pp. 39-61). Thousand Oaks, CA: Sage.

Root, M. P. P. (1997). *Filipino Americans: Transformation and identity.* Thousand Oaks, CA: Sage.

Rumbaut, R. G. (1995). The crucible within: Ethnic identity, self-esteem, and segmented assimilation among children of immigrants. In A. Portes (Ed.), *The second generation* (pp. 119-170). New York: Russell Sage.

Sodowsky, G., Kwan, K. L., & Pannu, R. (1995). Ethnic identity of Asians in the United States. In J. Ponteretto, M. Casas, L. Suzuki, & C. Alexander (Eds.), *Handbook of multicultural counseling* (pp. 123-154). Thousand Oaks, CA: Sage.

Strobel, L. (1994). The cultural identity of third-wave Filipino Americans. *Journal of the American Association for Philippine Psychology, 1*, 37-54.

Sue, D., & Sue, D. (1988). *Counseling the culturally different: Theory and practice.* New York: Wiley Press.

Tompar-Tiu, A., & Sustento-Seneriches, J. (1995). *Depression and other mental health issues: The Filipino American experience.* San Francisco: Jossey-Bass.

Wolfe, D. (1997). Family secrets: Transnational struggles among children of Filipino immigrants. *Sociological Perspectives, 40*, 457-482.

doi:10.1300/J015v30n03_06

Seeking Emotional Parity in Marital Relationships: A New Identity Challenge for Chinese Immigrant Women

Irene Chung

SUMMARY. This article discusses the emotional dimension of identity development among Chinese immigrant women: their emergent needs for attention, validation, and support from their spouses. Using this author's private practice experience with this population, the article illuminates the sociocultural reality of a group of Chinese immigrant women, and the therapeutic approaches that supported them in creating new meanings and options in their seemingly unsolvable dilemmas. doi:10.1300/J015v30n03_07 *[Article copies available for a fee from The Haworth Document Delivery Service: 1-800-HAWORTH. E-mail address: <docdelivery@haworthpress.com> Website: <http://www.HaworthPress.com> © 2007 by The Haworth Press, Inc. All rights reserved.]*

KEYWORDS. Emotional identity development, Chinese immigrant women

---

Irene Chung, PhD, is Associate Professor in Social Work, Hunter College School of Social Work at The City University of New York.

Address correspondence to: Irene Chung, Hunter College School of Social Work, CUNY, 129 E. 79th Street, New York, NY 10021 USA (E-mail: ichung@hunter.cuny.edu).

[Haworth co-indexing entry note]: "Seeking Emotional Parity in Marital Relationships: A New Identity Challenge for Chinese Immigrant Women." Chung, Irene. Co-published simultaneously in *Women & Therapy* (The Haworth Press, Inc.) Vol. 30, No. 3/4, 2007, pp. 75-85; and: *Feminist Reflections on Growth and Transformation: Asian American Women in Therapy* (ed: Debra M. Kawahara, and Oliva M. Espín) The Haworth Press, Inc., 2007, pp. 75-85. Single or multiple copies of this article are available for a fee from The Haworth Document Delivery Service [1-800-HAWORTH, 9:00 a.m. - 5:00 p.m. (EST). E-mail address: docdelivery@haworthpress.com].

Available online at http://wt.haworthpress.com

doi:10.1300/J015v30n03_07

Chinese immigrant women have a relatively short history in the United States. Prior to the passage of the Immigration and Naturalization Act of 1965, Chinese immigrants in the U.S. have been predominantly men who came as laborers, merchants, and professionals. Very few Chinese women were able to join their spouses or fathers in the U.S. due to anti-Chinese immigration legislations (Segal, 2002; Uba, 1994). Since the 1970s, the large number of Chinese women who have emigrated either as children or adults primarily from China, Hong Kong, and Taiwan, has finally equalized the Chinese gender ratio in this country (Segal, 2002). Those who come from China tend to be of lower socioeconomic background, while women who come from Hong Kong and Taiwan tend to be better educated and more proficient in English. Despite their differences in background and levels of acculturation, the majority of Chinese immigrant women work outside of their homes to supplement their households' income. Those who are married tend to continue to identify with the core traditional Chinese gender values of being self-sacrificial in the interests of their families as well as serving as the primary caretaker in the household (Bradshaw, 1994; Segal, 2002; True, 1990).

Literature about Chinese immigrant women often highlights the arduous task of straddling the demands of work and family in the U.S. as a major stressor in their lives. Their core struggle is depicted as similar to the experience of immigrant women from other collective cultures, specifically around being caught between their ethnic cultural value that emphasizes fulfillment of familial obligations and the reality of seeking career advancement in a competitive and individualized Western society (Bradshaw, 1994; Segal, 2002; True, 1990; Uba, 1994). For these women, this dichotomy of Asian and Western values is further complicated by the need to identify with and support their families in dealing with issues of discrimination and racism as immigrants of minority status, which must take precedent over their embracement of Western feminist ideals (Bradshaw, 1994; Chin, 1994).

While gender role conflicts and ethnic identity issues continue to be a valid source of stress for Chinese and other Asian immigrant women, there seems to be another dimension to these conflicts that is emerging as some of these women immerse further in the acculturation process. As a private practitioner working primarily with the Chinese immigrant population for the past fifteen years, this author has worked with an increasing number of women who sought consultation regarding their relationship with their spouses. While the issues and experiences of these women are by no means representative of those of their female compatriots, their emotional quagmires are indicative of the unique sociocultural reality of a group of Chinese immigrant women and speak to the importance of recognizing the varied paths of female identity development process among women of color. In providing an account of their therapeutic process and the intervention approaches used by this author, this article seeks to elucidate some of the challenges for practitioners in working with women of color as minority members of American society.

EMOTIONAL IDENTITY CRISIS

The emotional conflicts experienced by this group of Chinese immigrant women can be viewed as the challenge they face in consolidating old and new cultural values, and developing new bicultural identities (Bradshaw, 1994; Huang, 2003). Helms (1985) indicates that cultural-identity development is an all-encompassing process that includes "shifts in attitudes involving cognitive, affective, and cognative components" (p. 241). Thus, the emergence of emotional needs is an intrinsic component of a new identity formation. Traditionally, Chinese women were socialized to be submissive and docile as wives, yet capable and self-reliant as caregivers of the household. These seemingly contradictory role expectations often resulted in asymmetrical relationships that were void of emotional communication between Chinese women and their spouses, in contrast to the strong attachment ties these women developed with their children and their female peers (Dien, 1992). The process of immigration and acculturation apparently reinforces the women's relational gains and their strong attributes within and outside of the household. Thus, it is only a matter of time before the issue of emotional disparity with their spouses surfaces to the forefront.

Family Background and Presenting Problem of Clients

There are many background commonalities among these Chinese immigrant therapy clients. These are women who grew up in traditional Chinese families where "the parent-offspring relationship reigns supreme, and conjugal closeness is totally submerged" (Dien, 1992). Like their mothers, they married at an early age with little or no dating experience. Their married lives revolved around raising their children and, at the same time, working outside the home to supplement the family income. Their spouses, similar to their fathers, are traditional patriarchal males who are authoritative and emotionally aloof in their interactions within the family, and apparently also exhibit personality difficulties with management of their temperaments. The presenting problem of these women, however, was not about the burden of their multiple roles, which they actually perceived as an accomplishment and a source of pride. They generally viewed their problem as feeling "confused" about the quality of their spousal relationship, and they expressed concern that they sometimes became enraged with their spouses.

Help-Seeking Behavior

In their initial sessions, these clients were often hesitant about acknowledging the extent of their unhappiness with their relationships. Many of them came in initially to seek services for their children who had been affected by the lack of parental accord in the family. As these women became engaged with the worker to discuss the progress of their children and the family dynamics, they gradually disclosed some details of their interactions with their spouses. Their common comments were:

> I just want him to listen to me. He is never interested in having small talks with me.
>
> He always blames me when there is a problem with the children.
>
> I can never go to him if I am upset or worried about something.
>
> He always questions my decisions, and he always has to be right about everything.
>
> He always reminds me that he is a good husband because he is making more money and paying for most of the bills. To him, providing for the family is the criterion of a good husband.

With some discomfort, these clients talked about their interactions with other men on the job, and their observations of couple interactions and relationships portrayed in the media, which seemed "more desirable" than relationships with their spouses. Consequently, their first questions after such disclosure were invariably about whether their perceptions were "accurate," and if so, were they "being selfish" or "asking too much from their spouse?"

When this author validated their concerns, these clients were often quick to point out that they have often antagonized their spouses by ignoring their requests or making angry comments. Even in cases where they suspected that their spouses were involved in extra-marital affairs, they often expressed guilty feelings that they sometimes refused to have sex with their husbands, and asked for affirmation that their behavior did not precipitate the affairs.

Perception of Solutions to Problem

The second phase of the counseling sessions generally focused on the women's interest in taking steps to work on their relationships. They asked for this author's input in understanding the dynamics in their marital relationship, as well as suggestions on how to approach their spouses when they needed support and attention. As the sessions progressed and it became clear that their spouses lacked the insight and the capacity to make changes in their relationships, the women were faced with the task of reconciling the realities of their transformed emotional identity and being married to men who were unable to meet their emotional needs. As befitting the Chinese cultural values and norms, the possibility of pursuing a divorce was never in the forefront of their discussions. Some of them acknowledged that they had fleeting thoughts of leaving their spouses, but stated that they could not fathom the possibility of giving up their obligation to provide a family for their children. They regarded giving up their commitment to the marriage in pursuit of their personal happiness as a serious breach of their integrity, which would be regarded with shock and disapproval by their kinship network in the U.S. and in their home country. A few of them disclosed that in the past they had developed close friendships with men they encountered on the job, but ended the friendships when they realized that they were becoming romantically attached to these men. Most importantly, all of the women also expressed feelings of concern and attachments for their spouses as partners and family members who have gone through many trials and tribulations together in building their lives in the U.S.

The final phase of the counseling sessions was generally marked by these women's efforts to create some positive meaning of their circumstances and a sense of hope and direction in moving on with their lives. Having attempted to improve their relationships with their spouses and initiate more quality interactions, these women felt both vindicated and empowered. Reviewing their progress in taking control of their lives became a recurrent theme in the sessions. In their discussions, they were able to give themselves credit for promoting the welfare of their families. More importantly, they took pride in having made strides in their emotional gains. Through the process of their counseling sessions, many of these women came to the realization that they harbored feelings of fear toward their spouses that were similar to their sentiments toward their authoritative fathers in their childhood. Looking back, they recalled their mothers' acquiescent behavior around their fathers, and their own feelings of intimidation in seeking attention from their fathers. These women acknowledged that it was these historical feelings of fear that used to paralyze them from asserting their needs with their spouses. The dissipation of their fears toward their spouses, as these women took action to address the issues in their relationships, was a major contributing factor to their feelings of hope as they looked to the future.

As they gained insight and validation about their strengths and vulnerabilities from a historical perspective, these women also were able to make minor changes in their daily lives which alleviated some of their stressors and gave them a sense of personal space and control. Some of them took small vacations with their female friends or siblings after careful deliberation and making alternative child-care plans. Others eliminated some non-essential chores that they normally performed for their spouses. Such acts of asserting their self-interest with their spouses, who were deemed as fearful figures of authority at one time, denoted significant psychological changes for these women and, in turn, triggered positive repercussions in the family dynamics. Their spouses, sensing their wives' unhappiness and realizing the resources and opportunities available in American society for these women to leave their marriage, accepted the changes and even made some attempts to express their appreciation of their wives' support. The children, witnessing less stress in their mothers and less tension in the family, performed better in school and required less supervision at home. To these women, their success in bringing about family cohesion was a major validation of their role and a top priority in their schema of cultural constructs of well-being.

DISCUSSION

The Process of Emotional Identity Development

Discussants and researchers on the cultural-identity development of ethnic minority individuals generally agree that an individual's questioning and confusion about her identity, as precipitated by changes in the environment, is a crucial indicator that the individual is ready to explore and shift her internal views of self in relation to others (Helms, 1985). Regarding the Chinese immigrant women who sought counseling from this author, their work experiences afforded them an opportunity to be exposed to the Western ideal of emotional parity between men and women. In addition, their new status as gainfully employed members of American society offered them a sense of acceptance into the host culture and an opportunity for further acculturation. This new frame of reference regarding their perception of self and others invariably led to a reexamination of the nature of a marital relationship that had always been deemed as the norm in their family history. Given the core traditional values of these clients, which emphasize collectivity and interdependence (Segal, 2002; Uba, 1994), such questioning denotes a drastic shift in placing one's personal interest over others. It is understandable, then, that these clients initially discussed their issues in counseling sessions with discomfort and uncertainty, and would only seek consultation from a professional rather than their female peers. Since seeking professional counseling is commonly viewed as a stigmatized practice and a drastic departure from the traditional norms of help-seeking in the Chinese culture (Segal, 2002; Uba, 1994), these women's strength and courage in pondering changes in their lives should be noted.

By the same token, these women's attempts to own their responsibility for the problems of their marital relationships should be examined in the context of their cultural background which promotes the virtues of self-sacrifice and self-reliance among females (Dien, 1992). While one may conclude from a Western psychodynamic perspective that these women's behavior is an internalization of their problems and an indication of their low self-esteem, it is important to take into consideration their cultural and gender-specific constructs of well-being, which are significant motivational forces underlying those behaviors. Zastrow and Kirst-Ashman (1997) defined self-esteem as "a person's judgment of his or her own value" (p. 124). This personal judgment is, in essence, an internalized benchmark that is acquired through the individual's social and cultural norms. Researchers indicate that there are markedly divergent and culturally-specific behavior and goals between individuals of Asian and Euro-American cultures in their definition of self-concepts and emotional well-being (Markus & Kitayama, 1994; Oishi & Diener, 2001). In the Chinese collectivistic culture, behavior that conveys modesty, agreeableness, and sensitivity in anticipating the needs of others is deemed as socially desirable. Thus, positive self-esteem and the associated emotions need to be viewed as a subjective experience that is acquired through "the attainment of culturally prescribed goals, or engagement in culturally appropriate behavior" (Oishi & Diener, 2001, p. 1675).

Among this group of Chinese immigrant women, their aforementioned behavior can be viewed as culturally congruent and reflective of their strength and persistence in the face of hardship. While questioning and accepting their role in perpetuating their spouses' insensitive and domineering behavior, these women understood that having traditional parents from the old world as marital role models was a major factor that contributed to their confusion and "naiveté" in this matter. They were able to empathize with their mothers' passivity in tolerating relationships that were void of emotional support, and to draw parallels between their mothers' preoccupations with survival issues for their families during extended periods of war, poverty, and political unrest in China (Chin, 2000), and their own struggles with supporting their families after their immigration to this country. In this author's opinion, their ability to view their problems objectively from a trans-generational perspective and their willingness to attempt to resolve their issues demonstrated an intrinsic sense of self-confidence and positive self-esteem.

Finally, the Chinese immigrant women's emotional quagmires and their unwillingness to leave their spouses need not be viewed as failures on their part to acquire a more positive emotional identity. From a multicultural and feminist perspective, cultural-identity formation that involves gender role and emotional development may not follow a linear and prescribed course (Chin, 1994; Huang, 2003). Bradshaw (1994) posited that Asian immigrant women face many more political, economic, and psychological barriers in following the Western feminist ethos of "maximizing personal achievement" (p. 91). Due to their oppressed status as females and minority members of society, and the generally incongruous value orientation between middle-class American culture and the traditional Asian culture, these women often have to either embrace the White middle-class feminist values and risk losing the support of their family and indigenous community, or become further marginalized in the host society if they choose to remain in an emotionally oppressive environment. Such diametric choices, however, do not seem to afford the opportunity for genuine self-actualization. The challenge for these women, then, is to be able to create options and make changes progressively in their lives that are meaningful for them.

Therapeutic Approaches

As Constantine, Greer, and Kindaichi (2003) aptly pointed out, the transformation trajectory of women of color should be supported around the "synthesis of their own internal visions of womanhood" (p. 44). To facilitate this goal, it is crucial to develop a therapeutic relationship that conveys sensitivity to and acceptance of these women's unique and complex sociocultural reality, as well as their interpretation and creation of solutions. In working with Chinese immigrant women, this author utilized an eclectic host of approaches framed by a postmodern position that legitimizes "plurality, complexity, diversity, and the unremittingly contextual nature of human functioning" (Applegate, 2000, p. 146). On a cognitive level, this author provided clarification and sanction to these women's troubled emotions in response to their spouses' behavior. General knowledge about relationship and family dynamics and the historical impact of parent-child relationships were offered to these women to elicit their insights and connections in regard to their own life circumstances and family histories. On an intersubjectivity level, this author tried to be attuned to the feelings of these women and used herself differentially to respond to their specific emotional needs. Generally, their emotions ranged from feelings of uncertainty, embarrassment, and anger, to pride, relief, and hopefulness. In making specific emotional connections with these women, this author also attempted to be sensitive to when they were ready to discuss their feelings, and when they merely wanted some unspoken acknowledgement of their emotions. On a self-object level, this author played various transferential figures on cue from these women. These included serving as an advisor who dispensed strategies, but also elicited their input and improvisations; an authority figure who provided validation of their strengths, and yet accepted their ambivalence and vulnerabilities in their interactions with their spouses; and a patient listener who provided a venue for their emotional distress without dispensing advice and judgment. Such varied roles reinforced the empowerment of these women to seek the support they needed in forging their destinies in the midst of a seemingly unsolvable sociocultural dilemma.

CONCLUSION

Saari (1993) discussed the concept of identity as a complex meaning system that evolves from an individual's various domains of social experiences. As changes in life circumstances challenge the individual's perceptions and beliefs, it is important that the individual amends the different facets of her meaning system, so that "the content will fit with the context and experience of the present" (p. 17). The experiences of the group of Chinese immigrant women who sought counseling from this author illuminated their attempts to create meaning around an aspect of their lives that created conflict for them as a result of their acculturation into American society. From a post-modern perspective, the focus of clinical treatment is not so much about eradicating the causes of the client's problem, but rather supporting the client in the creation of "a more adequate meaning system . . . within which the client can make behavioral choices and cope with his or her current life" (Saari, 1993, p. 13). Thus, the outcome of these women's treatment should be credited with the relative coherence that they managed to create among their modified identity systems, as well as their enhanced capacity to retain options and behavioral choices in a bicultural milieu. Their accomplishment is, in essence, a celebration of multiculturalism and feminism.

REFERENCES

Applegate, J. S. (2000). Theory as story: A postmodern tale. *Clinical Social Work Journal, 28*, 141-153.

Bradshaw, C. K. (1994). Asian and Asian American women: Historical and political considerations in psychotherapy. In L. Comas-Diaz & B. Greene (Eds.), *Women of color* (pp. 72-113). New York: Guilford Press.

Chin, J. L. (1994). Psychodynamic approaches. In L. Comas-Diaz & B. Greene (Eds.), *Women of color* (pp. 194-222). New York: Guilford Press.

Chin, J. L. (2000). Mother-daughter relationships: Asian American perspectives. In J. L. Chin (Ed.), *Relationships among Asian American women* (pp. 119-132). Washington, DC: American Psychological Association.

Constantine, M. G., Greer, T. M., & Kindaichi, M. M. (2003). Theoretical and cultural considerations in counseling women of color. In M. Kopala & M. A. Keitel (Eds.), *Handbook of counseling women* (pp. 40-52). Thousand Oaks, CA: Sage.

Dien, D. (1992). Gender and individuation: China and the West. *Psychoanalytic Review, 79*, 105-119.

Helms, J. E. (1985). Cultural identity in the treatment process. In P. Pedersen (Ed.), *Handbook of cross-cultural counseling and therapy* (pp. 239-245). Westport, CT: Greenwood Press.

Huang, L. N. (2003). An integrative view of identity formation: A model for Asian Americans. In E. P. Salett & D. R. Koslow (Eds.), *Race, ethnicity and self* (2nd ed., pp. 37-53). Washington, DC: NMCI Publications.

Markus, H. R., & Kitamaya, S. (1994). The cultural construction of self and emotion: Implications for social behavior. In S. Kitayama & H. R. Markus (Eds.), *Emotion and culture* (pp. 89-130). Washington, DC: American Psychological Association.

Oishi, S., & Diener, E. (2001). Goals, culture, and subjective well-being. *Personality and Social Psychology Bulletin, 27*, 1674-1682.

Saari, C. (1993). Identity complexity as an indicator of health. *Clinical Social Work Journal, 21*, 11-24.

Segal, U. A. (2002). *A framework for immigration: Asians in the United States*. New York: Columbia University Press.

True, R. H. (1990). Psychotherapeutic issues with Asian American women. *Sex Roles*, 22 (7/8), 477-486.

Uba, L. (1994). *Asian Americans: Personality patterns, identity, and mental health*. New York: Guilford Press.

Zastrow, C., & Kirşt-Ashman, K. (1997). *Understanding human behavior and the social environment*. Chicago: Nelson-Hall.

doi:10.1300/J015v30n03_07

Asian American Women and Suicide: Problems of Responsibility and Healing

Eliza Noh

SUMMARY. Recent data on the alarming suicide rates among Asian American women are directing increasing public attention to this important mental health issue. However, very little is known about Asian American women's suicides from the perspectives of Asian American women themselves. This study examines the narratives of Asian American women suicide survivors about problems of responsibility for the purpose of therapy or healing. In particular, the study examines the role of individually focused healing therapies that seek to adjust the individual to society without questioning the power of racial and sexual subjection in hindering contexts for healing. As a result of a lack of language for suicide that moves beyond binarist discourses of victimhood or re-

Eliza Noh, PhD candidate, is Assistant Professor of Asian American Studies at California State University, Fullerton.

Address correspondence to: Eliza Noh, Asian American Studies Program, H-312E, California State University, Fullerton, 800 N. State College Blvd., Fullerton, CA 92834-9480 (E-mail: enoh@fullerton.edu).

[Haworth co-indexing entry note]: "Asian American Women and Suicide: Problems of Responsibility and Healing." Noh, Eliza. Co-published simultaneously in *Women & Therapy* (The Haworth Press, Inc.) Vol. 30, No. 3/4, 2007, pp. 87-107; and: *Feminist Reflections on Growth and Transformation: Asian American Women in Therapy* (ed: Debra M. Kawahara, and Oliva M. Espín) The Haworth Press, Inc., 2007, pp. 87-107. Single or multiple copies of this article are available for a fee from The Haworth Document Delivery Service [1-800-HAWORTH, 9:00 a.m. - 5:00 p.m. (EST). E-mail address: docdelivery@haworthpress.com].

Available online at http://wt.haworthpress.com

doi:10.1300/J015v30n03_08

covery, suicidal Asian American women are forced into silence about their psychic traumas or to represent their pain in self-destructive ways. The article suggests a rethinking of psychotherapy and healing that acknowledges the complex coexistence of agency and "illness," as well as the need for empowering Asian American women to change their sociopolitical environments. doi:10.1300/J015v30n03_08

KEYWORDS. Suicide, Asian American women, racism, sexism, healing

Recent data on the alarming suicide rates among Asian American women are directing increasing public attention to this important mental health issue. The Centers for Disease Control and Prevention have published statistics demonstrating that suicide is the second leading cause of death among Asian American women aged 15-24 (Centers for Disease Control and Prevention, 2003) and that Asian American women aged 15-24 and over 65 have the highest female suicide rates across all racial/ethnic groups (National Center for Health Statistics, 2003). Furthermore, Asian American adolescent girls (G5-12) demonstrate the highest rates of depression across both race/ethnicity and gender (Schoen, Davis, Scott Collins et al., 1997). In California, these statistics have prompted the State Assembly to proclaim May as API Mental Health Awareness Month in 2003.

While raising consciousness about this data is crucial, very little is known about Asian American women's suicides due to the scarcity of empirical studies on the subject, particularly from the perspectives of Asian American women themselves. Studies of suicide as a sociocultural phenomenon among Asian American women (Ibrahim, 1995; Miranda, 1992; Takahashi, 1989; Uba, 1994; Yu, Chang, Liu, & Fernandez, 1989) cite multiple factors, such as social alienation, depression, acculturation difficulties, trauma, racism, and sexism, as contributors to suicide. However, among these factors, the psychological impact of racism and minority status on Asian Americans, in general, is under-researched (Hall, Okazaki, & Nagata, 2002; Young & Takeuchi, 1998). Although studies may briefly recognize the "psychosocial stressors" of racism and sexism by failing to center sociopolitical factors, they inevitably pinpoint the individual or ethnic culture as the root of suicide or mental illness. The absence of a thorough critique of gender and racial trauma in these studies only serves to reinforce individually focused perspectives that ignore the significance of social structural inequalities in the creation of "mental pathologies." In *Mortality, Immortality and Other Life Strategies*, Zygmunt Bauman (1992) states, "The conscience of death is, and is bound to remain, *traumatic*" (p. 13). I take Bauman's analysis of trauma to mean the ways in which the social specter of death haunts the suicide, including the everyday reality of racism and sexism that threatens to kill the spirit and body. Root (1992) demonstrates that the destructive effects of racism, as well as heterosexism and classism, can be experienced by women as a form of insidious trauma that builds over time. However, within an individually focused framework, the *social* pathology of everyday racism and sexism becomes naturalized as "rational" or "normal." As a result, individually focused therapies seek to repair the individual psyche, instead of addressing systematic oppressions that are themselves pathological. Individually focused therapies are defined as therapeutic practices that rely on psychological theories and models that locate the source of psychic conflict, as well as the focus of change, within the individual. If traditional psychological theories and psychotherapies reflect primarily Western social and cultural philosophies (Bradshaw, 1994; Chin, 1994; Chin, 1998; Espín, 1994), then it can be argued that these therapies are informed by Western ideals that emphasize individualism, both in terms of focusing on the individual as the source of conflict (Butler, 1985) and unit of analysis (Chin, 1994; Comas-Díaz & Greene, 1994; Hall et al., 2002), and individuation or individual change as therapeutic outcome (Bradshaw, 1994; Espín, 1994).

This article examines the narratives of Asian American women suicide survivors about problems of responsibility for the purpose of therapy or healing. In particular, the article examines the role of individually focused healing therapies that seek to adjust the individual to society without questioning the power of racial and sexual subjection in hindering contexts for healing. As a result of a lack of language for suicide that moves beyond binarist discourses of victimhood or recovery, these Asian American women are forced into silence about their psychic traumas or to represent their pain in self-destructive ways. This article suggests a rethinking of psychotherapy and healing that acknowledges the complex coexistence of agency and "illness," as well as the need for empowering Asian American women to change their sociopolitical environments.

STUDY BACKGROUND

This article presents a portion of a larger study that examines how American women of Southeast Asian, East Asian, and South Asian descent experience suicide in relation to racial and sexual subjectification. Using original empirical research about suicide survivors, the study employs interdisciplinary methods of discursive and historical analyses of Asian American women's narratives in order to contextualize suicide within a sociopolitical framework. The research comprises interviews with 26 Asian American women, from college-age to their 50s, living in three major geographical areas of the US–San Francisco/Bay Area, Houston and New York. The study inquires about their suicide attempts and suicidal behaviors and thinking. The majority of the women interviewed represented the entire age range of the 20s, and totaled 15 in number. The breakdown of other ages is as follows: 6 adult teenagers, 3 in their 30s, 1 in her 40s and 1 in her 50s. As for ethnic breakdown, the study sample included 10 Chinese Americans, 4 Korean Americans, 3 Filipina Americans, 2 hapas or mixed-race Asian Americans, 2 transracial adoptees from Korea, 2 bi-ethnic Asian Americans (1 Chinese-Japanese and 1 Filipina-Chinese), 1 Indian American, 1 Vietnamese American, and 1 Japanese American. The actual composition of the geographical locations is more complex because although I interviewed women in the San Francisco/Bay Area, New York and Houston, many of them had previously moved from places that they considered more socially influential during their formative years. The following is the precise geographical breakdown: 10 from SF/Bay Area, 7 from Houston, 4 from New England/East Coast cities, 2 from Southern or Central California, 2 from Hawaii, and 1 from the Midwestern heartland. While quantitative studies of Asian American suicide are needed, this study attempts to contribute to Asian American suicidology, first, through an in-depth, qualitative examination of suicide narratives, and secondly, by demonstrating how racism and sexism influence Asian American women's suicides. However, since the topic of the larger study is beyond the scope of this article, this essay will focus on suicide narratives that deal with problems of race, gender, therapy, and healing.

THE PROBLEM OF RESPONSIBILITY

To integrate an understanding of suicidal subjectivity as both a product of socialization and an agent of healing, I suggest an examination of

Asian American suicide through the trope of "responsibility." Elizabeth Alexander's (1994, p. 91) question, "What do a people do with their history of horror?" is important in a consideration of racial trauma or terror in suicide subjectification because it reminds us first to think about the problem of responsibility–which, broken down etymologically, may be interpreted as the ability (or inability) to respond–before we begin to consider the possibility of representing trauma or recovery. What *do* we do with our histories of horror? That is, assuming we are not already so damaged as a result of trauma, or are still experiencing trauma on a regular basis that we are unable to find our tongues. Do we want to respond by representing our pain? Are we concerned that representation may never be enough to "correspond" with the pain, or that it may maintain the opening of our wounds? Are we not already doomed to represent the pain anyway? These are questions that must be considered before exploring ways to represent the suicide's racial trauma for the purpose of recovery. The idea of responsibility in healing also acknowledges the diverse range of abilities that Asian American women develop to address gender and racial traumas, from traditional therapies to alternative, individual, and communal acts of agency. Moreover, responsibility stresses social accountability and the necessity of transforming oppressive racialized and gendered relations of power to create social contexts for healing.

In order to examine questions of responsibility, I turn to Wendy Law-Yone's novel *Irrawaddy Tango* (1993), which thematizes the costs of representing psychic trauma. The text's response to trauma is fiercely anti-historical and anti-political, as well as anti-commemorative, as a result of the protagonist's simultaneously conditioned inability and refusal to participate in civilized conventions of responsibility. *Irrawaddy Tango* is an account of everyday terror, which Taussig (1992) similarly calls, "terror as usual." Departing from an elaboration of torture that relies on a separation between civilization and domestic safety on one side and worldlessness and pain on the other (Scarry, 1985), *Irrawaddy Tango* compels us to consider torture's dynamic as an everyday occurrence. If everyday objects of civilization can be made to disappear through torture's conventional strategies of inversion, then what is the status of torture in situations where terror, and its routine disappearance from social analysis, *is* the everyday–except an unusual epistemology of pain that forces us to reexamine altogether our ability to respond to the world. What would it mean to create an account of horror then?

Law-Yone's novel asks important questions about responsibility that should precede a practice of therapy and healing, such as how to deal with the difficulty of representing trauma, the problem of healing within oppressive contexts, and perhaps the impossibility of recovery itself. Many of the women I interviewed also raised these issues, in terms of their silence about their suicide attempts and their experiences of racial and sexual violence; the inescapability of their traumas, manifested through bodily self-mutilations and recurring memories of psychic pain; their resistance to traditional mental health services; and their rejection of easy narratives of healing. Bulhan (1985) argues that a psychology of oppression should address these issues:

> Why, for instance, do the oppressed manifest high resistance and suspicion when confronted with seemingly innocuous research questions? Why do they fail to take advantage of health services even as they admit a dire need for medical care? How can one explain the high drop-out rate observed among those of them who seek therapy? Why is it often so difficult to arrive at a correct diagnosis regarding maladies of the oppressed? And even when they are correctly diagnosed, why do such patients deliberately subvert the very prescriptions that would restore their health? (p. 11)

A Report of the Surgeon General (U.S. Dept. of Health & Human Services, 2001) confirms the prevalence of these issues, in particular for Asian Americans, who possess the lowest rates across gender, age, and geographic location for utilization of mental health services compared to other ethnic populations.

Reflecting these outcomes, the majority of the interviewees possessed either negative or ambivalent attitudes towards mental health services rather than positive experiences of therapy, in a ratio of almost two to one. For example, Lydia,[2] a Korean American woman in her early 20s, discusses her distrust of therapy's authoritative claims to objectivity:

> I don't really need a shrink. . . . Perhaps I can get hooked on a shrink or psychiatrist. . . . I think I do a good job of psychoanalyzing myself on a daily basis, let alone *pay* somebody to psychoanalyze me, who can be *completely* wrong about what I am.

Besides the dependency that psychoanalysis seems to cultivate, Lydia objects to the commodification of psychic care, especially among those with few financial resources. Interviewee Vicki, a woman of Chinese and Japanese descent in her 30s, similarly draws a connection between medical discourses and commodification:

> This seems to be a really, I guess, recent phenomenon of people deciding that it's a biochemical thing, and I think . . . that it's more cultural and it's also kind of *capitalistic*, because of marketing Zoloft and Prozac and all that. I think also it starts to become a middle-class phenomenon, maybe. It's just like eating disorders; you *can* have an eating disorder when you have the *means* to have one. It seems to be a really masturbatory, self-involved kind of thing. . . . And somehow that seems to be an easy *out*, so this friend of mine who defines herself as being a depressed person who can be cured by taking Zoloft, and I think there's something kind of fucked about that. First of all, it's defining yourself that way; then it's kind of a foregone conclusion. Second, relying upon pharmaceutical companies to cure you of some supposed ill. If you're saying, "I'm a depressed person," then that's *it*, "I'm just a person who's depressed," and it's like, "So you're a person who's depressed, but there's other things, too, like maybe it would help if you thought of yourself as a person who responds to stimuli in a certain way, and if you changed your response to stimuli, you would no longer fit into that category of a depressed person."

Vicki criticizes the circular logic that is contained in the labeling and treatment of clinical depression. Michel Foucault (1988) noticed that a similar circular logic characterized psychoanalysis in nineteenth-century European asylums:

> The science of mental disease, as it would develop in the asylum, would always be only of the order of observation and classification. It would not be a dialogue. . . . It would be fairer to say that psychoanalysis doubled the absolute observation of the watcher with the endless monologue of the person watched–thus preserving the old asylum structure of non-reciprocal observation but balancing it, in a non-symmetrical reciprocity, by the new structure of language without response. (pp. 250-251)

Thus, a new practice of managing pain and containing deviance was dissimulated through another enlightened discourse of rationality. However, this was not just a problem of European modernity. Psychoanalytic theories continue to be entrenched in American therapies (Schnog, 1997), even in spite of attempts to radicalize psychoanalysis and to correct the power imbalance inherent in the monological, confessional structure of psychotherapy:

> Although feminist, Marxist, and cultural critics have challenged the liberatory possibilities of a therapeutic practice marked by racial stigmas, class privilege, gender bias, and social myopia, such critiques and movements have not always succeeded in extirpating Freudian concepts from their own theories of group empowerment. This is particularly evident in the case of women's consciousness-raising groups, which rejected Freud's domestic reading of female nature (and his ever-loathed theory of "penis envy"), while incorporating his method of talk and self-confession as their baseline tactic for their remaking of the social order. To remodel psychotherapy as a "radical therapy" is still to envision radical politics within the conceptual frame of therapeutic talking cures. (p. 7)

The apparent difficulty of transforming psychotherapy's "talking cure" is one of the factors in its failure as an effective healing tool. As interviewee Janelle, a Chinese Canadian in her 20s, observes, "I think Western psychology–there's just no mystery to it. It's always the Freudian thing. It's always, 'What happened is the cause of this', and it's always the same conclusions, and I think I never had much trust in it, because it seemed so sterile to me."

The distrust of psychotherapy that Janelle describes is not uncommon among the suicide narratives because of power dynamics built on social stereotypes of Asian American women as passive, malleable creatures. In particular, the prevalence of the model minority ideology serves to discipline unruly Asian American subjects that disrupt the American myth of meritocracy and progress. P. W., a Chinese American woman in her late 50s, describes how her psychiatrist pathologized the distrust that she felt towards the larger society:

> [My therapist] saw my *distrust* of people as pathological. *Now* I don't see my distrust of people as pathological, *I see it as reality* . . . . I think a *lot* of how they saw pathology in me had to do with the whole model minority syndrome. The fact that I veered from what they felt was a *norm*, I think, really made it easy for them to see pathology in me. I think certainly the *psychiatrist* I was with

> was *more than willing* to see pathology. He gave me *all the drugs* for manic depressive illness.

P. W.'s experience demonstrates how the mental health system can help to enforce conformity by pathologizing individuals and disregarding structural oppressions, silencing them with clinical labels and pharmaceutical drugs. The result of this trend in the praxis of psychology is the systematic disempowerment of those in need of care from seeking healing strategies that attempt to change their social contexts:

> The fact that the vast majority of all our difficulties in life stem from oppression is ignored. The fact that we can reach out into our environments and change them is also downplayed and ignored. The fact that thousands of people are suffering in very similar ways from the structure of society is also ignored. We are discouraged from talking to each other, speaking out, organizing, etc. (Re-evaluation Counseling Communities, 1991, p. 57)

In some cases, the psychological counseling professions not only discount the reality of oppression and fail to support proactive efforts to resolve problems, but also directly contribute to the mental anguish of their patients by invalidating their perspectives and substituting them with their own. Marine, a hapa[2] in her late 20s, illustrates the violation of trust she experienced with her psychiatrist:

> I've had experiences with psychiatrists that have been fucked up. There was one psychiatrist who realized I worked at this one good company, and she said, "Is it OK if I mentioned your name so my friend could inquire about a position there?" I was like "yeah," and then the next thing I know the human resources person says, "I know she's your doctor, but she keeps on calling me." So that was very scary. The other psychiatrist that I found very difficult–she truly was very difficult. She was passing moral judgments on my lifestyle. Like about my sexuality, like about racism. She was a white woman, so she just thought that I was being very uppity and difficult and making things more than they were. So she just said, "Come on, it's not like that." And she'd say, "I don't think that's what it means," and "Are you sure that's what you should be doing?" She was like, "I find you very difficult, and the kind of medication you are on, you are bipolar anyway, so obviously you're going to be very violent." And she starts using my illness against

> me, and she starts saying, "It's obvious you're going to act this way because you're sick anyway."

As exemplified in Marine's case, the individualization and invalidation of women's traumas often have to do with the illegibility of the oppressions that Asian American women experience. As discussed earlier, the terror of everyday racism and sexism seems simply to disappear from social analysis because terror and its social ignorance are so integrated into our "civilized" cultural thinking. As a result, women like Andie, a Korean American trans-racial adoptee in her 20s, are forced to second-guess the reality of racist oppression since there does not seem to be a legitimate language for it: "I think it *did affect me*, that subtle kind of racism that you can't really pinpoint because they're not *saying* anything wrong." Similarly, Jill, a Japanese American woman in her 30s, describes the lack of accountability for everyday racism and its damaging, cumulative impact on her psyche:

> It's always difficult to articulate, because there is nothing you can directly point to. . . . These minor incidences of racism, I think they accumulate over time. So it's often hard to point to one incident. Point to one person. But it gave you this kind of sense of yourself through these small incidences that say, "Well, maybe I'm not good enough. I'll never be good enough. I always have to measure up to these other people." And if I do call it out, then there's certain ramifications I really have to think hard about before I do, . . . like people getting angry over the race issue at me or . . . trying to accommodate it and sometimes not even in the right ways. . . . But that still doesn't erase institutionalized racism across the board.

As Jill relates, efforts to speak up about racism usually result in racist backlash, whether to make claims of "reverse discrimination" or offer accommodating concessions. Meanwhile, institutional racism continues unrecognized, pushing women like Jill into a marginalized position of either stigmatization or pathological silence and self-blame.

Many Asian American women remain silent about their psychic suffering in order to avoid compounding it through abuses by the mental health system. Lydia, for instance, did not attempt to seek care after she overdosed on pills. She explains:

> The reason why I didn't want to go to the hospital was because I knew that regardless they were going to ask me about my health

> insurance situation or whatever. I just knew that I don't really want to go to the hospital because I can't afford it. And if there was anything about like, oh, they would bring in the child protective services or whatever, like I knew that it was shitty to be in my family, but I knew that it would be even shittier if I *wasn't* in the family. Just in terms of physically being transplanted to a foster home or something. And I didn't want that, so I didn't really tell anybody.

Lydia represents one of many Asian Americans who lack the financial resources to afford appropriate health services, which seems to be more and more prevalent in America's HMO/insurance company-driven health-care system. On another institutional level, Lydia must face the additional obstacle of social services, which only serve to alienate her further by trying to remove her from her only place of familiarity. Lydia describes an instance when she could not seek help for herself because she felt she was forced to choose between her family and the social work system:

> I hate the social work system. This is after my brother hit me pretty bad. I was pretty messed up in high school. They took me out of class, and this social worker came from the child protective services, and he said that I'd have to go to a foster home . . . the *approach*, logistically in how they *come* and *bombard* your whole house and system, I'm really not for that. You're not going to sit there and conform to this *White* family like they wanted me to; they wanted to send me to some *White* family. A, I already have White people issues, and B, I'm not going to sit there and be like, "OK, Mom, they're going to put you under questioning, while I'm sitting here thriving in some affluent, *White* family." I wasn't for that either.

While some women that I interviewed did seek the help of social services, they usually saw it as a last resort and tended to have ambivalent attitudes toward the system because of its lack of cultural understanding and sensitivity about their home situations. In the instance that Lydia describes above, the inappropriateness of the social work approach extends beyond a cultural insensitivity about Asian Americans' tendency to stress family cohesion and reluctance to speak out about personal or private issues. The social work system failed to take into account the impact of racism on this family. It placed Lydia in an impossible position of dividing her family, labeling it as "pathological" in contrast to the White foster family. With her use of the word "bombard," Lydia indicates an antagonistic relationship between her family and institutional authorities. Other women I spoke to also objected to the forced nature of counseling and social services:

> Janice (19-year-old Chinese American): I remember one time in the middle of it, this other nurse said, "Okay we're going to have this social worker come talk to you. And did you know it's a federal crime to commit suicide in the state of California?" and something like, "It's against the law to kill yourself." And I thought that was totally ridiculous.

> Andie: . . . It was forced counseling. The way it was explained to me was that it's illegal for somebody to try to kill themselves, and so when you're a minor, it means you either have to go into a mental hospital or you have to go through counseling once a week. So that's what I did, and the counselors were kind of worthless.

As Janice's and Andie's experiences illustrate from the perspectives of individuals in pain needing care, it seems surprising that there would be a penal aspect in the treatment of suicide attempts. This raises the question of the policing function of mental health care, according to Supeene (1990): "Psychiatry is the only branch of medicine that expects to force treatment on people and which can invoke the aid of the police to do so" (p. 73). In cases of mistreatment through the mental health system, it is no wonder, then, that Asian American women develop a distrust of these social institutions.

As a result of a lack of social resources, those Asian American women who have experienced traumas must continue to suffer in silence and learn to suppress their psychic pain as a means of coping. Lydia says about her painful experiences, "I think a lot of it has been suppressed for so long that why even bring it out? I've just been so used to not telling anybody things that it just comes to me second-nature not to say anything. And just like history, you can be selective in what you want to tell people." Lydia creates self-denial about her pain, but as she explains in the following passage, her silence also functions as a survival mechanism:

> Do you know in my lifetime, I never once said that I was depressed, which is weird. . . . Guilt and depression are two highly paralyzing emotions for me because you can't do anything about

> it. . . . For me personally, things have been *bad*, but at the same time, I was always busy *hiding* the fact that it was bad that sometimes I wouldn't even think that it was bad. . . . I think the reason why I don't tell people is because I don't want them to view me in a different way, and perhaps it's very deceiving and whatever, but that's really how I look at things. I don't want them to, A, feel pity or whatever, *or* feel like, "You've overcome so much adversity. You persevered in life." I don't really want to hear that either. If anything, it was just like a survival method, like this is what you do in order to get where you want to be.

Lydia echoes the perspectives thematized in *Irrawaddy Tango*, in which the female protagonist rejects self-disclosure due to discourses of containment implicit in public confessions. Perhaps Lydia uses her silence and, to an extent, her denial to deal with the lack of understanding and empathy that exists socially, particularly within the dualistic social discourses that she describes, which offer only two modes of expressing injury–either victimhood or recovery.

As in *Irrawaddy Tango*, many of the women I interviewed confronted problems of responsibility, or of representing their pain. They found speaking about their suicide attempts either impossible or insufficient to express their psychic pain, so their traumas became inscribed instead through their physical bodies. Sometimes the women consciously inflicted physical self-abuse. For example, Gabrielle, a Korean American in her late 20s, often strangled or hit herself. Soyeon, another Korean American in her late 30s, attempted suicide three times, as well as abused drugs and alcohol. During her second attempt, she burned her own hands in boiling water so severely that she required surgery. She feels that she burned herself to show her pain and anger in a physical way because of her suppressed feelings. Sometimes psychic pain exhibited itself psychosomatically, as in the back and neck pains of twenty-something Chinese American Laney. In other cases, pain registered through a combination of intentional or unintentional physical acts of self-destruction. Mindy, a Filipina in her mid-twenties, cut her wrists and experienced anxiety attacks, eating disorders, and breakdowns that manifested physically as well as emotionally. P. W. suffers from asthma and agoraphobia, which she believes are related to many years of stifled self-expression and confinement. She also developed a nervous facial twitch, which she believes resulted from her childhood anxiety about speaking only English. Vicki expressed her suicidality not by attempting suicide, but by placing herself in physically dangerous or risky situations: abusing drugs, hitchhiking with strangers, having indiscriminate sex, and cutting herself with razor blades. Rachael, a twenty-something Korean American adoptee, showed several physical manifestations of suicidal tendencies: chronic migraine headaches, agoraphobia, and alcohol and drug abuse, explaining that "it was like, 'maybe I could just O.D'." As in Rachael's case, addiction was prevalent among the suicidal women.

Among the physical acts of self-mutilation, cutting or scratching seemed to be most common. For instance, in addition to abusing alcohol, Marine attempted suicide twice by slashing her wrists. Gabrielle, Jerry, and Hayley, a 19-year-old Korean American, all describe cutting or scratching themselves with blades, pins, or their own fingernails. For some women, like Gabrielle and Jerry, self-abuse was an expression of anger that they directed towards themselves. In addition to abusing drugs and alcohol, Asha, a 19-year-old Indian American, regularly cut her arms with razors, scissors, and needles, which she says was due to unexpressed anger from having to "hide everything." Vicki explains that cutting herself was like having "an intense bodily experience" that she could not express verbally: "Being able to articulate my feelings wasn't something that I was raised to do and so it just was very gratifying, and it's like this real tangible thing." Similarly, Jill believes the idea of cutting herself made her pain more real:

> It seemed so attractive to kind of feel the pain. Like my last willful act to actually be able to feel something because I was totally not able to feel anything at that point or very little. . . . Just putting the knife to my wrist, going through the motion in my head, was some kind of *release* in a way. . . .

Both Jill and Janice, who cut her arms and legs with pins, describe feelings of release, as if physically cutting themselves offered a kind of relief of pent-up internal pain. In Gabrielle's case, her psychic experience was made real not only through the feeling of pain, but by the resulting physical wounds, like a hieroglyphics of the flesh that would display and legitimize her pain:

> It was like a visible reminder to me, and maybe half-wanting people to see it as well. I think it helped me to feel some of the things that I wasn't allowed to feel. Or things I couldn't talk about. So it just kind of made my angst real for me, since I could say, "It *hurts*."

By manifesting their psychic states physically, the women's experiences speak to a problem among Asian American women of articulating trauma and of suicidal agency. For Jill, feeling the sharp pain of cutting represents a final willful act within her otherwise numb existence. In this sense, the body responds, expressing pain where words fail. For Vicki, however, ultimately taking her own life would require agency that she feels she did not possess:

> I didn't even feel that I had enough ownership of my own self to say, "Okay, I'm going to kill myself," because I didn't feel like I could *do* that, like I even had that much authority over my own self to do that. Sometimes that's the *one* agency that you feel that you have, and I think I actually didn't feel I even had that. . . . I have this belief that the power over your own existence is the *most* power that you can have, and maybe that was why I couldn't embrace suicide, because I didn't feel that I had the sanction to have that kind of power, and I didn't ultimately act. That is the *one* most *defining* act of power, is to kill yourself.

Vicki describes a feeling of suicidal abjection that maintains her trauma's illegibility and ultimately her silence. Except for a series of reactive, self-destructive behaviors, subjective agency fails to materialize through words or through bodily inscriptions, foreclosing the possibility of response-ability or healing.

IMPLICATIONS

These narratives about suicide and healing demonstrate problems of therapies that individualize psychic traumas. Focusing on individuation as a therapeutic outcome is particularly problematic for Asian American women whose sources of identity and support may be found in their ethnic communities and families. Furthermore, by focusing solely on individual or intrapsychic conflicts and ignoring sociopolitical causes of Asian American women's suicides, particularly racial and gender oppressions, these therapies hinder effective healing contexts. As anti-racist and feminist therapies demonstrate, health and illness must be understood as emerging out of ever-present social contexts of racism and sexism (Bair & Cayleff, 1993a; Espín, 1994). Without necessary validation of their individual experiences as being connected with larger social forces, Asian American women deal with problems of responsibility, or of representing their pain through silence, self-blame, and self-destruction. But also expressed in these narratives of self-destruction are moments of agency, through the women's desire to maintain authentic responses to their pain, whether by rejecting easy narratives of recovery or expressing pain through non-verbal means. Therefore, it is necessary to move beyond binarist conceptualizations of healing by recognizing the complex and sometimes contradictory subjectivities within suicidality. The coexistence of illness and agency suggests that an Asian American feminist approach to healing cannot be found within the cult of the individual, where a unitary conceptualization of self-healing translates into the goal of recovery and wholeness, but rather in the adaptive realities of ambivalence that Asian American women actually live. For Asian American women, maintaining ambivalent feelings, such as anger, about their colonized mentalities can be seen as a strategy of resistance against colonization, instead of as pathology (Bradshaw, 1994; Comas-Díaz, 1994). Moreover, within a social context where the "pursuit of happiness" is ideologically hegemonic and antithetical to the reality of suffering, the therapeutic goal of achieving happy wholeness can create problems (Bradshaw,1994) of guilt and inadequacy for Asian American women who do not fit this image. The pressure of letting go of any feeling that does not conform to the stereotype of the meek and mild model minority is particularly salient for Asian Americans who are always expected to assimilate and not make waves.

Moving beyond individualist approaches to healing and taking into account social context mean that we may need to rethink the role of psychotherapy, including those emphasizing "culturally sensitive" approaches. Most therapies concerning Asian Americans focus on cultural differences or advocate cultural sensitivity (Bradshaw, 1994; Chin, 1998). Culturally sensitive models address the need to challenge the Eurocentric (as well as androcentric) focus of psychotherapy, and of psychology in general, which, as some have argued, are inappropriate for diagnosing and treating Asian Americans (Chin, 1998; Homma-True, 1997). Notwithstanding the importance of cultural competence in psychotherapy, I believe that there is a bias toward viewing Asian Americans through a culturalist lens due to contradictory racial ideologies prevalent in the US that continually objectify Asian Americans as cultural others and, at the same time, ignore their subjectification as racial others. Moreover, culture is over-emphasized and race de-emphasized in regards to Asian Americans for the same reason that race is over-emphasized and culture de-emphasized in regards to Black Americans, which has to do with how each group has been socially managed throughout US racial history (Chin, 1994). For example, Asian Americans are commonly racialized as immigrants, whose cultural status, i.e., their ability or inability to assimilate or acculturate, always seems sufficient to explain their existence in the US, resulting in social stereotypes preoccupied with their cultural assimilation, such as the "model minority" or the "perpetual foreigner." (Whereas, Black Americans are racialized not as immigrants, but as slaves or property lacking in cultural history, so that only their skin color or "race" seems important.) While some Asian American psychologists have called for an analysis of race and minority status, along with culture (Chin, 1998; Hong & Domokos-Cheng Ham, 2001; Sue, 2002), relatively little research has actually addressed race and the sociopolitical context (Hall et al., 2002). As a result, Asian American feminist therapy risks creating what Bair and Cayleff (1993b) call a "new cultural relativism" or "the danger of becoming so immersed in ideas of cultural difference that the political and socioeconomic origins of illness . . . are overlooked" (p. 89). Another danger of cultural relativism is the tendency to view culture in static terms and to culturally objectify Asian Americans as always different or other. Rooted in Western racial perspectives about Asian Americans, psychotherapies that focus on acculturation, assimilation, and conformation to mainstream cultural values as therapeutic outcomes should be called into question as hegemonic strategies of social control (Bradshaw, 1994; Chin, 1994; Chin, 1998). Therefore, it may be useful to combine an analysis of racial and gender ideologies with analyses of culture when counseling Asian American women.

My own empirical research, which demonstrated that Asian American women suicide survivors employed diverse healing strategies from traditional therapies to alternative practices (cultural decolonization through writing and art, spirituality, social activism, and Asian medicine–the details of which are beyond the scope of this essay), seems to suggest that healing models must be flexible enough to accommodate therapeutic as well as extra-therapeutic interventions. While anti-racist and feminist therapy have drawn attention to the impact of racism, colonialism, and sexism in psychology, and suggested ways to modify traditional therapy to be less Euro- and andro-centric, I think that revisionist therapies are limited and more radical approaches are necessary, especially when it comes to matters of life and death as in suicide intervention. Comas-Díaz (1994) asserts that for women of color, therapy should be nothing short of a process of "psychotherapeutic decolonization," by affirming racial and gender identity, self-determination, and autonomous dignity. Chin (1998) similarly argues that mental health services need to move beyond the perspective of Asian Americans as a group that needs to be accommodated, through modifying current models to creating delivery systems based on ethnic-specific principles. There is much room for ethnic and cultural specificity since most therapists continue to be trained in theories that are Western- and male-oriented, and even feminist scholarship on mental health and health care continues to focus on the experiences of White, middle-class women (Bair & Cayleff, 1993a; Bradshaw, 1994; Comas-Díaz & Greene, 1994a; Espín, 1994). If "feminist therapists acknowledge that therapy per se is not a cure-all" (Butler, 1985, p. 37), then they should be mindful of their own myopic gaps and take seriously the healing power of transforming the social context beyond therapy. When working with Asian American women, this entails providing extra-therapeutic support services, such as advocacy and information, fostering community networks, and encouraging social action and empowerment (Bair & Cayleff, 1993; Bradshaw, 1994; Chin, 1998; Comas-Díaz, 1994; Espín, 1994; Lee, 1997). The therapeutic relationship itself should be a bottom-up rather than a top-down dialogue, in which the therapist evaluates issues on a case-by-case basis through active listening and taking cues from the client in an attempt to put aside monolithic stereotypes about Asian American women (Bradshaw, 1994; Comas-Díaz, 1994). This dialogue is also critical, given the low utilization rate of mental health services among Asian American women. Moreover, it should lead psychotherapists to pay attention to the usefulness of diverse responses to healing, rather than simply trying to get Asian American women to accept conventional therapy. Ultimately, it may be that achieving mental well-being cannot be found simply through psychotherapy, but by making necessary changes in the sociopolitical environment and creating new, empowering forms of subjectivity that draw from the unique experiences of Asian American women.

NOTES

1. All subjects' names used are pseudonyms.

2. The term hapa refers to Asians or Pacific Islanders of mixed ethnic or racial heritage. Marine identifies as Filipina, Chinese, Mexican and European.

REFERENCES

Alexander, E. (1994). Can you be black and look at this?: Reading the Rodney King video(s). *Public Culture, 7*, 91-110.

Bair, B., & Cayleff, S. E. (1993a). Introduction. In B. Bair & S. E. Cayleff (Eds.), *Wings of gauze: Women of color and the experience of health and illness* (pp. 13-17). Detroit, MI: Wayne State University Press.

Bair, B., & Cayleff, S. E. (1993b). Traditional medicine and holistic concepts of health: Questions of culture and politics. In B. Bair & S. E. Cayleff (Eds.), *Wings of gauze: Women of color and the experience of health and illness* (pp. 89-92). Detroit, MI: Wayne State University Press.

Bauman, Z. (1992). *Mortality, immortality and other life strategies.* Palo Alto, CA: Stanford University Press.

Bradshaw, C. K. (1994). Asian and Asian American women: Historical and political considerations in psychotherapy. In L. Comas-Díaz & B. Greene (Eds.), *Women of color: Integrating ethnic and gender identities in psychotherapy* (pp. 72-113). New York: Guilford Press.

Bulhan, H. A. (1985). *Frantz Fanon and the psychology of oppression.* New York: Plenum Press.

Butler, M. (1985). Guidelines for feminist therapy. In L. B. Rosewater & L. Walker (Eds.), *Handbook of feminist therapy* (pp. 32-38). New York: Springer.

Centers for Disease Control and Prevention (2003). Deaths: Leading causes for 2001. *National Vital Statistics Reports, 52*(9), 1-86.

Chin, J. L. (1994). Psychodynamic approaches. In L. Comas-Díaz & B. Greene (Eds.), *Women of color: Integrating ethnic and gender identities in psychotherapy* (pp. 194-222). New York: Guilford Press.

Chin, J. L. (1998). Mental health services and treatment. In L. C. Lee & N. W. S. Zane (Eds.), *Handbook of Asian American psychology* (pp. 485-504). Thousand Oaks, CA: Sage.

Comas-Díaz, L. (1994). An integrative approach. In L. Comas-Díaz & B. Greene (Eds.), *Women of color: Integrating ethnic and gender identities in psychotherapy* (pp. 287-318). New York: Guilford Press.

Comas-Díaz, L., & Greene, B. (1994). Overview: Gender and ethnicity in the healing process. In L. Comas-Díaz & B. Greene (Eds.), *Women of color: Integrating ethnic and gender identities in psychotherapy* (pp. 185-193). New York: Guilford Press.

Espín, O. M. (1994). Feminist approaches. In L. Comas-Díaz & B. Greene (Eds.), *Women of color: Integrating ethnic and gender identities in psychotherapy* (pp. 265-286). New York: Guilford Press.

Foucault, M. (1988). *Madness and civilization: A history of insanity in the age of reason.* New York: Vintage Books.

Hall, G. C. N., Okazaki, S., & Nagata, D. (2002). Epilogue: Toward the future of Asian American psychology. In G. C. N. Hall & S. Okazaki (Eds.), *Asian American psychology: The science of lives in context* (pp. 195-200). Washington, DC: American Psychological Association.

Homma-True, R. (1997). Asian American women. In E. Lee (Ed.), *Working with Asian Americans: A guide for clinicians* (pp. 420-427). New York: Guilford Press.

Hong, G. K., & Domokos-Cheng Ham, M. (2001). *Psychotherapy and counseling with Asian American clients: A practical guide.* Thousand Oaks, CA: Sage.

Ibrahim, F. A. (1995). Suicidal behavior in Asian-American women. In S. Canetto & D. Lester (Eds.), *Women and suicidal behavior* (pp. 144-156). New York: Springer.

Law-Yone, W. (1993). *Irrawaddy tango.* New York: Alfred A. Knopf.

Lee, E. (1997). Overview: The assessment and treatment of Asian American families. In E. Lee (Ed.), *Working with Asian Americans: A guide for clinicians* (pp. 3-36). New York: Guilford Press.

Miranda, N. (1992). *The rising suicide rate among Asian American youth.* Unpublished master's thesis, Columbia University School of Journalism, New York.

National Center for Health Statistics (2003). *Health, United States, 2003.* Hyattsville, MD: US Public Health Service.

Re-evaluation Counseling Communities (1991). *What's wrong with the "mental health" system, and what can be done about it.* Seattle, WA: Rational Island Publishers.

Root, M. P. P. (1992). The impact of trauma on personality: The second reconstruction. In L. S. Brown & M. Ballou (Eds.), *Personality and psychopathology: Feminist reappraisals* (pp. 229-265). New York: Guilford Press.

Scarry, E. (1985). *The body in pain: The making and unmaking of the world.* New York: Oxford University Press.

Schnog, N. (1997). On inventing the psychological. In J. Pfister & N. Schnog (Eds.), *Inventing the psychological: Toward a cultural history of emotional life in America* (pp. 3-16). New Haven, CT: Yale University Press.

Schoen, C., Davis, K., Scott Collins, K., Greenberg, L., Des Roches, C., & Abrams, M. (1997). *The commonwealth fund survey of the health of adolescent girls.* Retrieved April 25, 2004, from http://www.cmwf.org/programs/women/adoleshl.asp

Sue, S. (2002). Foreword. In G. C. N. Hall & S. Okazaki (Eds.), *Asian American psychology: The science of lives in context* (pp. xi-xiii). Washington, DC: American Psychological Association.

Supeene, S. L. (1990). *As for the sky, falling: A critical look at psychiatry and suffering.* Toronto, Canada: Second Story Press.

Takahashi, Y. (1989). Suicidal Asian patients: Recommendations for treatment. *Suicide and Life-Threatening Behavior, 19*(3), 305-311.

Taussig, M. (1992). *The nervous system.* New York: Routledge.

Uba, L. (1994). *Asian Americans: Personality patterns, identity, and mental health.* New York: Guilford Press.

U.S. Department of Health & Human Services (2001). *Mental health: Culture, race, and ethnicity–A supplement to mental health: A report of the Surgeon General.* Rockville, MD: Substance Abuse & Mental Health Services Administration.

Young, K., & Takeuchi, D. T. (1998). Racism. In L. C. Lee & N. W. S. Zane (Eds.), *Handbook of Asian American psychology* (pp. 401-432). Thousand Oaks, CA: Sage.

Yu, E., Chang, C. F., Liu, W., & Fernandez, M. (1989). Suicide among Asian American youth. In M. Feinleib (Ed.), *Report of the secretary's task force on youth suicide* (pp. 157-176). Washington, DC: U.S. Department of Health and Human Services.

doi:10.1300/J015v30n03_08

Feminist Therapy: Its Use and Implications for South Asian Immigrant Survivors of Domestic Violence

Diya Kallivayalil

SUMMARY. Feminist therapy is a compelling framework to use with women who are survivors of domestic violence due to its focus on power and oppression in women's lives. However, feminist frameworks have been criticized for their lack of attention to the experiences of diverse

---

Diya Kallivayalil is a doctoral student in Clinical/Community Psychology at the University of Illinois at Urbana-Champaign and is currently doing her predoctoral psychology internship at Cambridge Hospital/Harvard Medical School. Her research and clinical interests include the impact of trauma, violence, sexual harassment, and migration on women's mental health, and patterns of psychopathology, emotion, and family socialization among immigrant families.

Address correspondence to: Diya Kallivayalil, Cambridge Hospital, Division of Psychology/Department of Psychiatry, 1493 Cambridge Street, Cambridge, MA 02139 (E-mail: kallivay@stat.psych.uiuc.edu).

This paper is based on a dissertation project being conducted by the author at the University of Illinois at Urbana-Champaign. This research was supported by the University of Illinois Research Board, the Marianne Ferber Dissertation Award from the Women's Studies Program at the University of Illinois at Urbana-Champaign, and the Bardwell Memorial Research Fellowship from Mount Holyoke College.

The author gratefully acknowledges the support and guidance of her advisor, Sumie Okazaki, and the insightful contributions of her dissertation committee members: Nancy Abelman, Nicole Allen, Manisha Desai, and Louise Fitzgerald. Her warmest gratitude to the practitioners who shared their thoughts with her.

[Haworth co-indexing entry note]: "Feminist Therapy: Its Use and Implications for South Asian Immigrant Survivors of Domestic Violence." Kallivayalil, Diya. Co-published simultaneously in *Women & Therapy* (The Haworth Press, Inc.) Vol. 30, No. 3/4, 2007, pp. 109-127; and: *Feminist Reflections on Growth and Transformation: Asian American Women in Therapy* (ed: Debra M. Kawahara, and Oliva M. Espín) The Haworth Press, Inc., 2007, pp. 109-127. Single or multiple copies of this article are available for a fee from The Haworth Document Delivery Service [1-800-HAWORTH, 9:00 a.m. - 5:00 p.m. (EST). E-mail address: docdelivery@haworthpress.com].

Available online at http://wt.haworthpress.com

doi:10.1300/J015v30n03_09

groups of women, a shortcoming that multicultural frameworks have attempted to address. Very little scholarship exists on the use of feminist therapy with South Asian women, and with Asian American women in general, particularly on its use with domestic violence survivors. The work that does exist suggests that Asian values are in contrast with the principles of feminist therapy for a variety of reasons. Using interviews with practitioners who work with battered South Asian women, this paper suggests that practitioners enact feminist and multicultural principles in their work, by their attention to sociocultural context, their focus on women's empowerment and voicing women's lived experiences, and their consideration of the dynamics of the therapeutic relationship. They hold patriarchy in its complexity accountable for domestic violence in the community. Although the term "feminist" was rarely used, in contrast to work that suggests that Asian women would not identify with self-based models of therapy, practitioners articulated that women do benefit from insight-based therapy, and attempted to work against cultural stereotypes that they often see functionally used to evade addressing trauma and grief. doi:10.1300/J015v30n03_09 *[Article copies available for a fee from The Haworth Document Delivery Service: 1-800-HAWORTH. E-mail address: <docdelivery@haworthpress.com> Website: <http://www.HaworthPress.com>*

KEYWORDS. South Asian, domestic violence, feminist therapy, culture, patriarchy, multicultural therapy

Feminist therapy is a compelling modality to use with women and children who are survivors of domestic violence, primarily due to its explicit focus on the influence of power and oppression in women's lives, and its location of pathology in patriarchy and other external factors that determine the domination and control of women (Sharma, 2001; Burstow, 1992). These very factors are held responsible for the pervasiveness of domestic violence as one of the many socially sanctioned forms of violence against women (Bishop, 1994; Burstow, 1992; Walker, 1979).

Apart from these core assumptions, the guidelines and goals of feminist therapy, as outlined by Sharma (2001), include close attention to sociocultural context, demystification and relative equalizing of the therapeutic relationship, and a focus on women's empowerment. Women are encouraged to draw on their strengths and coping abilities to make their own decisions and feel in control of their actions to protect themselves, and Sharma (2001) has recommended it as a beneficial and powerful form of intervention with domestic violence populations. This has also been borne out in certain empirical studies (e.g., McCloskey & Fraser, 1997).

Despite their strengths, feminist frameworks have been criticized for their minimizing of the true diversity of women's experiences, particularly with regard to race, ethnicity, migration history, sexual orientation, and religion, by their identification of gender as the focal point of oppression for women (Espín & Gawelek, 1992; Greene, 1994; Ho, 1990). Scholars have suggested that despite their commitment to draw on the experiences of all women, feminist models tend to overgeneralize from the experiences of White, western, middle-class women (Espín, 1994; Sharma, 2001). This also has specific clinical implications, as White therapists who may attempt to reconfigure the imbalances in the therapeutic relationship by examining their sexist assumptions may not have exercised the same reflection with regards to their racial or class-based assumptions (Brown, 1990; Sharma, 2001). Further, by not fully appreciating the structural barriers and oppressions that minority or immigrant women face, therapists may encourage women to leave an abusive relationship without realizing that this action might place women and their children at risk for deportation, among other issues (Macleod & Shin, 1990).

In contrast, multicultural frameworks for therapy have explicitly addressed the shortcomings of traditional forms of therapy with understudied and minority groups by calling attention to both the ethnocentrism of mainstream therapy and the special needs and issues of these groups (e.g., Sue & Sue, 1999). According to one perspective, the multicultural perspective is "defined as a philosophy that affords the development of flexibility and diversity in orientations to life and for the development of pluralistic identities" (Ramirez, 1983, p. 157). The assumptions behind this perspective include a focus on the strengths of different communities, the acknowledgment that we do not live in a color-blind society, that psychological reality is not fixed in time and space (or by one community), and a distancing from stereotypes (Cervantes & Cervantes, 1993). Further, scholars and practitioners of color have sought to reclaim and diversify feminist frameworks; Mays and Comas-Diaz (1988), for example, argue that as feminist philosophy has diversified and become more integrative, it has become more appealing to ethnic minorities.

CLINICAL INTERVENTIONS WITH ASIAN AMERICAN COMMUNITIES

While this paper addresses feminist interventions with South Asians most specifically (a group who claim their geographical heritage from India, Pakistan, Nepal, Bhutan, Bangladesh and Sri Lanka), much of the existing literature does not differentiate between subgroups of Asians in the United States. Therefore, the Asian American literature is discussed and work done with South Asians is mentioned wherever available.

Both the feminist and multicultural frameworks are relevant to and inform work with Asian American women. With growing numbers of ethnic-specific services and scholars examining therapeutic issues with Asian Americans, the literature indicates that Asian Americans (including South Asians) underutilize mental heath services, partly due to the stigma associated with mental health issues, and also because mental health providers are not sensitive to the cultural and linguistic needs of Asian American clients (Sue, 1993; Sue, Nakamura, Chung, & Yee-Bradbury, 1994). To address this underutilization, multicultural frameworks have addressed the shortcomings of mainstream Western therapeutic models and urge scholars to pay attention to the specificities of Asian American communities.

One important piece in the literature is the suggestion that the values of Asian communities are at odds with prevailing Western principles of therapeutic intervention. According to Sue et al. (1994), "Asian Americans may have culturally biased views of mental health and illness and appropriate sources of treatment that are inconsistent with Western views" (p. 63). Although less work has been done with subgroups of Asians, the work that has been done with South Asians suggests similar factors at play; in general, the Western model of individual psychotherapy can be alien to South Asians (Durvasula & Mylvaganam, 1994; Preisser, 1999). The literature suggests that therapeutic goals such as individual self-actualization and self-disclosure would "contrast with traditional Asian Indian perspectives of the ideal person" (Durvasula & Mylvaganam, 1994, p. 103), given that the importance of any particular individual in a family may be minimized. While it is important to critique Western-developed therapy models for their ethnocentrism, the current arguments tend to rely on broadly drawn dichotomies and characterizations of eastern and western ideologies of personhood. According to Ito and Maramba (2002):

> Most of the literature about the problems Asian American clients face with non-Asian American therapists is based on assumed differences in belief systems between western-based therapeutic practices and etiologies and minority clients' beliefs and interpretations of the meaning and treatment of mental illness. Existing literature on the beliefs of Asian Americans about psychotherapy is largely conceptual and rarely supported empirically. Furthermore, the conceptual discourse is organized around broadly drawn differences between eastern or traditional Asian beliefs and western or conventional psychotherapy beliefs, which often results in caricatures of opposition of cultural differences. (p. 34)

As we will see in the next section, similar characterizations are often used in the limited literature that exists on feminist therapy with Asian American women.

Feminist Therapy with Asian American Survivors of Domestic Violence

The existing research on domestic violence in the South Asian community continues to grow and there is excellent descriptive work that addresses the role of gender socialization and the interplay of ethnicity, class, and legal status with this population (e.g., Abraham, 2000; Dasgupta & Warrier, 1996). Abraham (2000) also examined organizational ideology (value-oriented, diffused and unspecified) among six South Asian women's organizations in the United States that work to end violence against women. Of these six, four of the organizations considered their orientation "explicitly feminist, with the struggle to end patriarchy seen as central" (p. 158).

However, there is no empirical body of research on the use of feminist *therapy* with Asian American women in general, or with specific subgroups (such as South Asians) under this large umbrella. Further, there tends to be some conflation of feminist theory and feminist therapy in the literature, as well as a conflation of social service or advocacy-based intervention and therapeutic intervention. This makes it considerably more difficult to identify the work on "clinical" intervention, if we can make this distinction at all. Keeping this in mind, the research on interventions that does exist is largely conceptual and addresses domestic violence interventions (not necessarily, though frequently, feminist in orientation) with women of color more generally. Papers frequently involve a description of the shortcomings of traditional therapeutic models for domestic violence with communities of color, and then offer subsections that briefly address the "culture-specific" features of various, broadly defined communities, such as African Americans, Native Americans, Hispanic Americans, and Asian Americans (e.g., Cervantes & Cervantes, 1993; Enns, 2004). Some themes in this scholarship suggest that feminist work can be inherently contradictory to "Asian" values, and cite the subordination of women in Asian families, their emphasis on power and its vertical distribution in families, and their collectivist orientation as both providing the context for domestic violence and as inhibiting to feminist interventions (Cervantes & Cervantes, 1993; Kim, 1985; Preisser, 1999).

More recent work by Asian American scholars has attempted to explain in a nuanced way the more concrete dimensions and factors within the Asian community that are relevant to feminist paradigms of domestic violence and represent a leap forward in terms of a multicultural and contextual view of intervention (e.g., Ho, 1990; Preisser, 1999; Yick, 2001). In her important essay addressing multicultural and feminist approaches to domestic violence, Ho (1990) encourages us to pay close attention to contextual issues that are relevant to Asian and other immigrant groups such as immigration history, linguistic unfamiliarity, social isolation, diversity within Asian groups, generational issues, and the experiences of racism in the United States, when conceptualizing and designing interventions. This attention to sociocultural context is one principle of feminist intervention (Sharma, 2001). Further, these issues are clinically critical in situations of domestic violence, because they shed light on the resources and choices that many Asian women, for various reasons, have at their disposal. Close attention to them may prevent therapists from pathologizing their responses and perspectives as dependency, lack of individuation, or being "slaves to culture."

In many ways, however, these works also suggest that "Asian culture" is incompatible with the assumptions and practices of both Western forms of therapy and with feminist interventions. This incompatibility arises primarily from issues of collectivism and individualism and the assumed vertical hierarchy of Asian families. For example, Yick (2001) cited Masaki and Wong (1997):

> Many Western mental health paradigms, for example, which focus on self-care and the individual, are dissonant with traditional Asian values, which emphasize the collective unit, such as the family. (p. 548)

More specifically, Ho (1990) suggested that the "traditional" Asian values of close family ties, hierarchy, and order may create a permissive or at least tolerant atmosphere for physical and verbal abuse in the home. She argued:

> Each member of the family is expected to keep harmony, adhere to a specified hierarchical role, and comply with familial and social authority to the point of sacrificing his/her own desires and ambitions. (p. 134)

She also cited the importance of filial piety, fear of "loss of face," the emphasis on self-restraint in behavior, and the perceived difference in behavior in private and public spheres as factors that are relevant to the rise of conflict in Asian families. Finally, she argued that domestic violence is rooted in the oppression and devaluation of women, and the rigid sex roles, particularly with regards to marriage, that are commonly seen in Asian communities.

Although less scholarship has been done on the use of feminist therapy among subgroups of Asian Americans, more work has occurred on the conceptual front, and similar factors (patriarchal socialization, rigid gender roles, primacy of the family structure) have been cited as relevant to Chinese American and South Asian families, and as factors that prevent battered women from these groups from leaving abusive relationships (Abraham, 2000; Yick, 2001). Although Yick argued that feminist theory has a lot to offer in terms of its focus on patriarchy as underlying the permissive context for domestic violence, she believes that it does not pay attention to the family context and cultural values that Chinese American women have to deal with. In other words, Chinese women may not identify with feminist values of empowerment, which may have implications for feminist intervention. She stated:

> Feminist theories on domestic violence emphasize values of empowerment and self-determination; however, these values may not be culturally congruent with Chinese values (Rimonte, 1991). When a Chinese victim of domestic violence does opt to leave the abusive relationship, in essence, she decides to place her well-being over that of the collective system (i.e., the family). As a result, feminist ideologies espousing self-determination, autonomy, and individualism may be dissonant with a Chinese woman's cultural values. (2001, p. 552)

Similarly, South Asian scholars also imply that the traditionalism with respect to gender roles in South Asian society comes from a long history of myths and traditions that prescribe a self-sacrificial and interdependent role for women (Goel, 2005). These implied indoctrinated gender roles make women less likely and less willing to embrace intervention that focuses on autonomy, assertion, and that is conducted outside the familiarity of the family unit. In writing on a non-therapy form of intervention (the restorative justice model) with South Asians, Goel said,

> Self-assertion, a modern feminist value, is seen as neither deeply rooted in Indian history nor as a natural result of evolution. Rather, such values are foreign and reflective of the imperialist colonial influence. A woman who puts her own needs first is a woman who has become European/Western, shameless, and not truly Indian. (2005, p. 656)

Similarly, Preisser (1999), in discussing models of intervention that focused on understanding "cultural values" for battered South Asian women stated, "However, we must recognize that most of these intervention methods are founded on interdependence and are compatible with a South Asian woman's understanding of self" (p. 692).

Whether or not these characterizations are considered useful or accurate representations of Asian communities (and certainly no one would deny that all communities, including the South Asian community, do indeed permit and enact patriarchy), they explicitly or implicitly suggest that Asian values and ways of being are not congruent with feminist ideologies, which sets up a contradictory tension between feminist therapy and Asian women. They may also suggest that Asian societies are uniquely patriarchal and that Asian women may themselves buy into patriarchy for "cultural" reasons. Further, there are dangers in implying that in leaving abusive relationships, women chose to place their well-being over that of the family. This may not be the most appropriate dichotomy in which to think of a woman's action as it could imply that the entire family opposes the woman being safe, that the children are also not being abused, and that women who leave are "choosing" to do so for their "well-being" and not for safety. It also suggests that "feminism" is an entirely western concept, which is not the case (see Mohanty, 1991, for a discussion of third world feminisms).

Although it is critical to outline the contextual, linguistic, and practical concerns of Asian and immigrant women who are survivors of domestic violence, and address these concerns in therapy (for a tabular representation of a variety of issues and types of abuse and perpetrators, see Preisser, 1999), an unabashed focus on this mode of intervention may promote the idea that these women would only respond to "practical approaches," and would not respond to or be capable of more self-based modes of therapeutic intervention. This approach is promoted by the perception that Asians prefer more directive and less insight-based forms of interventions (e.g., Huang, 1991; Okamura & Agbayani, 1991). Certainly, it would be extremely difficult to address these latter issues in therapy when a client's safety and basic needs are not addressed, but many recommendations for interventions do not promote a balance between the two.

Of course, when considering the use of feminist therapy with Asian American women, it does appear that much of the feminist therapy practiced in the United States is indeed based on a Western model, and I am not suggesting that a singular vision be imposed on these women, especially since the therapeutic relationship itself is overrun with issues of power and privilege. However, in the context of examining the implications of feminist therapy with South Asian survivors of domestic violence, though not necessarily as the "only way," it becomes difficult to do so critically when the background is overlaid with the assumptions that their "values" are incompatible. It is this background that needs examination.

PURPOSE OF THE CURRENT STUDY

One useful forum in which to examine these assumptions, on the levels of both conceptualization and therapeutic techniques, is to document the experiences of practitioners who work with South Asian survivors of domestic violence. A number of closely related questions helped me conceptualize these issues: Do practitioners enact principles of feminist and multicultural treatment with their South Asian clients? This practice may exist on dimensions of both conceptualization and intervention. In what ways is this enacted and how is it named? Do practitioners encourage empowerment, broadly defined, beyond the huge burden of "practicalities" that survivors of domestic violence face? How do they face the challenge of practicing a "Western" treatment model with a perhaps unwilling audience?

Perspectives of South Asian Practitioners

In-depth qualitative interviews were conducted with seven practitioners who work with South Asian women as part of an ongoing project studying the mental health consequences of domestic violence among women of South Asian origin in the United States. Recruitment of the participants was done through a mental health agency in a large metropolitan area that serves the South Asian community. They represented a variety of roles: psychiatry, social work, psychology, education, and advocacy and all were South Asian. Each practitioner worked closely with South Asian women who are in relationships where domestic violence is present, or who have mental health concerns as a result of domestic violence. Because each was part of a setting that was committed to providing culturally competent services to the South Asian immigrant community, the following analysis is more explicitly focused on the ways their approach reflects principles of *feminist* intervention and how practitioners negotiate the complexities of context.

Conceptualization

In differing ways, practitioners articulated a feminist notion that patriarchy is the root of domestic violence in the South Asian community (and society at large), though the word "feminism" was not often used. They believed that South Asian culture was excessively paternalistic and rigid in terms of gender stereotypes that were articulated to children starting from a very young age, and resulted in a lack of respect for women. With the added pressure of immigration and changing gender roles, patriarchy was more firmly rooted than ever. For example, one therapist said:

> There are stereotypes about men and women and how they should behave and be, starting from practices when they are very young. Now things are changing, I feel that it is kind of threatening to the male population, which has been brought up with the notion that they have to be the superior one and the other one is the inferior one, you know? So it kind of gets threatening to them, that there is someone who's becoming their equal and as a result of that, because they feel this kind of an inferiority, they try to show their old superiority by resorting to violence. Which might be physical, sexual, emotional, mental. Any form.

Other workers articulated a similar take on this notion, and illustrated how forms and manifestations of abuse were also tailored by these forms of patriarchy. For example, one practitioner talked about the challenges of getting the opportunity to talk openly about abuse with South Asian women, particularly when they did not necessarily see what they had experienced as sexual or reproductive abuse, and the impact of patriarchal "mentality" on family action. She said:

> So when they do come here [for another presenting issue], they come with their husbands, who will fill out the forms for them, who will answer questions for them. A woman in her 5th month [of pregnancy] wanted to know the sex of her child because she's had two previous abortions because once she finds out the sex of the child, it's always a female. So they didn't . . . the husband didn't want that, he only wanted a boy, it didn't matter how many abortions she had to go through or whatever the case was. He only wanted a son. Because the mentality is it's somehow the wife's fault [that] they're not having a boy.

In other words, therapists articulated their own view on patriarchy and the rights of women that they attempted to pass on to their clients. In addition to this, however, they were also very attuned to the specificities of familial and immigrant life (in other words, attention to sociocultural context, which is also considered a feminist principle) that may make the disclosure of abuse that much more complicated, such as living in small apartments with extended family and the cultural "acceptance" of extended family presence in private spaces such as bathrooms and bedrooms. For example, one practitioner talked about cases of incest:

> It could be an uncle [who is the perpetrator]. Or father's friend, a very close family friend where again, because the culture's a certain way, anyone your father or your mother ever introduces to you that's elder turns into an uncle or an aunt. So I hear stories about that and because the culture is so, that's something that's such a taboo, no one wants to talk about it. So the children never approach the parents. They never want to say it because they feel shameful. Somehow they think it's their fault. Like maybe they dressed a certain way, or they provoked it somehow, and some of that leads to rape. Because a female says no regardless, you know, and it doesn't have to be a verbal no, it can be a physical no, like pushing some-

> one away or flinching the body or you know, whatever, it's still a no and I think any action that happens after that is rape.

Intervention

On the intervention front, the primary concerns for women, as practitioners saw them, were financial dependence, lack of education, immigration issues, what would happen to their children both in terms of custody and raising them on their own, and shame of what people in their native country and in their current community would say. The practitioners saw the truth and significance of all of these concerns, as each had interacted with women who had been shunned by their friends, family, and community as a result of speaking out about abuse. Therefore, they focused very concretely on the lived experiences of women (Espín, 1994). Although social pressure was a real concern, therapists were committed to not just addressing women's acute symptoms and helping them negotiate the systems they were interacting with (their children's school, the courts, public assistance), but also to helping women discover an identity apart from or in addition to being a wife and mother, and be able to articulate safely their own needs and independence. The importance they placed on self-hood, self-esteem, and self-worth was poignant, and they believed that self-knowledge and decisions based on it may have been lost in the abusive marriage, but was a priority in therapy, and helped women make concrete and empowering future decisions, whatever they may be. One therapist said:

> My approach has been that I try to make women look inside themselves and find out exactly what they are most comfortable with. Get to that level. And to discover themselves. Discover their own identity, what they want to do. What is the situation that they would like to be in and then work towards that. So for example if someone wants to study or something like that, to find out, what do you want to study, how to go about it. Or if you want to be financially independent, or if you want to maybe be a better mother or something like that.

They also expressed that women did not necessarily resist the "Western" idea of therapy, and saw their relationship with their clinician as important and supportive. It was also the case that some women did not only want to discuss the "practical" or role-determined aspects of their marriage, but were willing to engage their feelings about relationships and intimacy. One therapist talked about a client who had been abused from the beginning of her marriage, in which both these issues arose: feelings of deprivation of a "loving and normal" conjugal relationship, and her attitude towards the demystified therapeutic relationship:

> Finally she came over here and she was severely depressed then. She was suicidal, you know, and she talked about, I didn't know actually I had this kind of privilege, like I could come to you [for therapy]. She said, my marriage, I don't know what is the bond or relation, the loving relationship with my husband, I don't understand those things, because I never had those kinds of relations with my husband.

An important aspect of doing such non-judgmental and supportive work, and a feminist principle as articulated by Sharma (2001), was having a deep understanding of the patience and process it took to work with survivors of domestic violence and a validation of each woman's choices, particularly when they were still in the abusive relationship. Therapists articulated that often women spent many months in therapy simply talking about the abuse because they finally had a willing and supportive audience, as well as going back and forth on decisions (which was also understood in the context of their legal and financial dependence). It was also the case that women would bring up the topic of abuse one week and refuse to discuss it the next. This was sometimes worrisome in a traditional therapeutic sense because they were not able to begin a treatment plan or use specific CBT techniques, but they recognized this as a critical part of the treatment plan for survivors of domestic violence, as well as a real challenge in therapy. One therapist said of giving voice to women who had been silenced:

> You know, she just keeps on coming maybe crying and talking, talking but maybe that is the first step, you know, that she wants. That she needs. To just remove everything out of her. And feel like someone has heard about all the pain that she went through. Because a lot of these women, they feel that they have very much been cheated, no one heard them. For example, maybe they tried to tell their families or they tried to tell their friends, whatever they tried to do, no one no one there to help them, to listen to them.

Therapists were thus committed to enabling women to tell the story of their lived experience. Further, they followed the principles of enabling women to recognize that the problem lies not with them but with the larger social structure, and encouraging them to value their own hopes and identity. They also employed various methods to empower their clients, while remaining flexible to each woman's situation, particularly as it related to immigration and safety. They also described that their commitment to their clients extended beyond the therapy session or meeting. One clinician described how she modified her involvement depending on the situation, but in the end left the decision to them after providing information on self-protection and empowerment.

> Actually it depends on the intensity of the you know, of how much they are victimized, if I see their life is in danger in that family, then I prefer them to, when an emergency happens they should call 911 and go to a shelter, something like that. Other than that you know, trying to, talking, educating them about the resources, how they can protect themselves, their children. Like, if I am comfortable that she can handle, because she didn't have that kind of education she didn't know that [the information], you know, I try to empower them, you know, how to handle the whole situation.

Some practitioners took an even stronger or more direct approach to empowerment and although they respected their client's choices, they were not wedded to a family maintenance model, even when there was intense societal pressure. If women did decide to stay in their marriages, therapists used their time with them to change their perspective on their role in the family and the sources of power they did have. One clinician described a client whom she encouraged to use the system to improve her living situation.

> He used to hit her day after day, he had feelings like she is not part of this family, she is like a servant over here, she came over here for cooking, cleaning and taking care of the children. And the husband starting hitting her . . . those in-laws, never tried to protect her, instead of doing that they also encouraged him to you know oh, abuse ladies. Then, she once got the courage to call 911. And police came and the case started and she came over here for the counseling. And after I saw her I think probably for 8 or 9 sessions and then once she told me, I want to withdraw this case. Then I said why? Once you get the courage to report, you have to give him some sort kind of punishment, so that he understands that you are you know, part of the family, where you are feeling that you are

> not. And like she said no, you know, the people are talking bad about me. I'm not respectful, I'm very ungrateful, so I don't want to come over here anymore. And an order of protection was issued against husband and he was outside of the family then. And she's you know, satisfied with the money he is sending to her, to support the family, for the children. She is satisfied with that. She is like, oh my husband, he is not living with me, still he is sending money, he is taking care of us, like doing grocery for the family. I said, this is his job, he has to do that. That doesn't mean he's changed him. You know, he is not hitting you anymore, it doesn't mean that. You have to have patience, you know, you have to give him a good lesson.

She therefore encouraged clients to be skeptical about change, and in this case, used the temporary (legal) power to ensure his changed behavior. Her words also implied that women sometimes get taken in easily by small changes, especially when husbands help them financially when they are in difficult straights, and see this as a larger change. She saw part of her role as letting her clients know that their husbands have responsibilities they should always fulfill.

Another therapist said that cultural competence, as she saw it, was about understanding the broad contextual differences between people of different communities, as promoted by both multicultural and feminist frameworks; for example, she believed that although South Asians do not talk about sexuality as openly, she also believed that being victims of trauma and abuse led to a common experience of suffering. "After, all," she said, "Pain is pain." She also said that as a therapist, patience was required to work with people of all groups, not just South Asians. When I asked her how she negotiates the perception that therapy may be "culturally dissonant" for South Asians, she said that although she has encountered that view (often from family members of the abused woman or child), "I group all those statements about the Western model and everything under resistance. Then I work through that." She told me how in one case, family members of a child who had been sexually abused try to influence her not to take the issue as seriously by telling her that she is Indian "just like them." In other words, although she acknowledged that people have affiliations to different cultural groups, she suggested they sometimes used these popular stereotypes to avoid confronting painful familial issues. Setting up a division between South Asia and America and blaming "Western" influences is an issue with mental health in the community more generally. According to Bopanna (2005), who has worked with South Asians with bipolar disorder:

> Sometimes, when the symptoms of bipolar illness are first presenting, there is a tendency to blame the ill person and their Western values, especially if they are second generation Americans, as the cause of the illness. Perhaps because the illness presented in America and there was no awareness of it back home in the South Asian countries, there is a tendency to see it as a result of living here. Conversely, sometimes the symptoms are seen as signs of Western values themselves rather than illness! (2005)

CONCLUSIONS AND RECOMMENDATIONS

These interviews illustrate that, on both levels of conceptualization and intervention, practitioners who work with the South Asian domestic violence population enact feminist and multicultural principles, in their attention to sociocultural context, their focus on women's empowerment and voicing women's lived experiences, and focus on the dynamics of the therapeutic relationship. They hold patriarchy in its complexity accountable for domestic violence in the community. Although the term "feminist" was rarely used, and in contrast to work that suggests that Asian women would not identify with self-based models of therapy, practitioners articulated that women do indeed benefit from making the personal political and from insight-based therapy. Therapists attempt to work against stereotypes about both South Asia and the "West" that they see as often functionally used to avoid addressing trauma and grief.

While this study contained the perspectives of South Asian practitioners, who may be more familiar with the larger issues that South Asians in the United States face, the consideration of context, and its impact on the therapeutic relationship, is something that should be prioritized by all therapists. By not giving in to a priori assumptions about the traditionalism of the South Asian community, and by identifying patriarchy in domestic violence situations instead of attributing them to "cultural values," all therapists can promote education on these issues. Many of the practitioners I spoke with also conduct workshops and group meetings on domestic violence in the larger South Asian community. In this way, they promote the re-thinking of gender issues with a wider audience, and also attempt to counter the stigma and silence on both the issues of domestic violence and mental health. On the therapeutic level, the frank consideration of patriarchal and structural issues in the community enables women to examine the external forces that contributed to their situation, rather than blame themselves for the abuse. Further, it is important for all therapists to understand the specific constraints and opportunities that battered South Asian women may face, and construct interventions that work around them. In this way, they can also facilitate women's deeper engagement with the therapeutic process by assisting them with practical concerns, but also by focusing on their own needs and identity to promote long-term healing. They can thus promote feminist therapy with a focus on empowerment, women's lived experiences and choices, and a commitment to multiculturalism, as feminist therapy is indeed a powerful intervention tool with diverse domestic violence populations.

REFERENCES

Abraham, M. (2000). *Speaking the unspeakable: Marital violence among South Asian immigrants in the United States.* New Brunswick, NJ: Rutgers University Press.

Bishop, A. (1994). *Becoming an ally: Breaking the cycle of oppression.* Halifax, Canada: Fernwood.

Bopanna, R. (2005, May). How do desis respond to bipolar disorder in their spouses and friends? *ABCD Lady,* 12-20.

Brown, L. S. (1990). Ethical issues and the business of therapy. In H. Lerman & N. Porter (Eds.), *Feminist ethics in psychotherapy* (pp. 60-69). New York: Springer.

Burstow, B. (1992). *Radical feminist theory: Working in the context of abuse.* London: Sage.

Cervantes, N., & Cervantes, J. (1993). A multicultural perspective in the treatment of domestic violence. In M. Hansen & M. Harway (Eds.), *Battering and family therapy: A feminist perspective* (pp. 156-174). Thousand Oaks, CA: Sage.

Dasgupta, S. D., & Warrier, S. (1996). In the footsteps of "Arundathi": Asian Indian women's experience of domestic violence in the United States. *Violence Against Women, 2*(3), 238-259.

Durvasula, R., & Mylvaganam, G. (1994). Mental health of Asian Indians: Relevant issues and community implications. *Journal of Community Psychology, 22,* 97-108.

Enns, C. (2004). *Feminist theories and feminist psychotherapies: Origins, themes and diversity.* New York: The Haworth Press, Inc.

Espín, O. M. (1994). Feminist approaches. In L. Comas-Diaz & B. Greene (Eds.), *Women of color: Integrating ethnic and gender identities in psychotherapy* (pp. 265-287). New York: Guilford Press.

Espín, O. M., & Gawelek, M. A. (1992). Women's diversity: Ethnicity, race, class and gender in theories of feminist psychology. In L. S. Brown & M. Ballou (Eds.), *Per-*

sonality and psychopathology: Feminist reappraisals (pp. 88-107). New York: Guilford Press.

Goel, R. (2005). Sita's trousseau: Restorative justice, domestic violence, and South Asian culture. *Violence Against Women. 11*(5), 639-665.

Greene, B. (1994). Diversity and difference: Race and feminist psychotherapy. In M. P. Mirkin (Ed.), *Women in context: Toward a feminist reconstruction of psychotherapy* (pp. 333-351). New York: Guilford.

Ho, C. (1990). An analysis of domestic violence in Asian American communities: A multicultural approach to counseling. In L. S. Brown & M. P. P. Root (Eds.), *Diversity and complexity in feminist therapy* (pp. 129-150). New York: Harrington Park Press.

Huang, K. (1991). Chinese Americans. In N. Mokauau (Ed.), *Handbook of social services for Asian and Pacific Islanders* (pp. 95-112). Orlando, FL: Academic Press.

Ito, K., & Maramba, G. (2002). Therapeutic beliefs of Asian American therapists: Views from an ethnic-specific clinic. *Transcultural Psychiatry, 39*(1), 33-73.

Kim, S. (1985). Family therapy for Asian Americans: A strategic-structural framework. *Psychotherapy, 22*(2), 342-348.

Macleod, L., & Shin, M. (1990). *Isolated, afraid and forgotten: The service delivery needs and realities of immigrant and refugee women who are battered.* Ottawa, Canada: National Clearinghouse on Family Violence, Health and Welfare.

Masaki, B., & Wong, L. (1997). Domestic violence in the Asian community. In E. Lee (Ed.), *Working with Asian Americans: A guide for clinicians* (pp. 439-451). New York: Guilford Press.

Mays, V. M., & Comas-Diaz, L. (1988). Feminist therapy with ethnic minority populations: A closer look at Blacks and Hispanics. In M. Dutton-Douglas & L. Walker (Eds.), *Feminist psychotherapies: Integration of therapeutic and feminist systems.* Norwood, NJ: Ablex Publishing.

McCloskey, K. A., & Fraser, J. S. (1997). Using feminist MRI brief therapy during initial contact with victims of domestic violence. *Psychotherapy, 34*, 433-446.

Mohanty, C. (1991). Under western eyes: Feminist scholarship and colonial discourses. In C. Mohanty, A. Russo, & L. Torres (Eds.), *Third world women and the politics of feminism.* Indianapolis: Indiana University Press.

Okamura, J., & Agbayani, A. (1991). Filipino Americans. In N. Mokauau (Ed.), *Handbook of social services for Asian and Pacific Islanders* (pp. 95-112). Orlando, FL: Academic Press.

Preisser, A. (1999). Domestic violence in South Asian communities in America: Advocacy and intervention. *Violence Against Women, 5*, 684-699.

Ramirez, M. (1983). *Psychology of the Americas: Mestizo perspectives on personality and mental health.* Northvale, NJ: Jason Aronson.

Sharma, A. (2001). Healing the wounds of domestic abuse: Improving the effectiveness of feminist therapeutic interventions with immigrant and racially visible women who have been abused. *Violence Against Women, 7*(12), 1405-1428.

Sue, D. W., & Sue, D. (1999). *Counseling the culturally different: Theory and practice.* New York: Wiley.

Sue, S. (1993). The changing Asian American population: Mental health policy. In LEAP Asian Pacific American Public Policy Institute and UCLA Asian American Studies Center (Eds.), *The state of Asian Pacific America* (pp. 79-94). Los Angeles: LEAP Asian Pacific American Public Policy Institute and UCLA Asian American Studies Center.

Sue, S., Nakamura, C., Chung, R., & Yee-Bradbury, C. (1994). Mental health research on Asian Americans. *Journal of Community Psychology, 22*, 61-67.

Walker, L. E. (1979). *The battered woman.* New York: Harper Perennial.

Yick, A. (2001). Feminist theory and status inconsistency theory: Application to domestic violence in Chinese immigrant families. *Violence Against Women, 7*(5), 545-562.

doi:10.1300/J015v30n03_09

Asians and Native Hawaiian or Other Pacific Islanders Midlife Lesbians' Health: A Pilot Study

Suzanne L. Dibble
Noriko Sato
Ellen Haller

SUMMARY. The purpose of this pilot study was to determine actual and potential health issues of midlife lesbians who were Asian American, Native Hawaiian, or other Pacific Islanders (A-NHOPI). We explored the health status (body composition, "outness," smoking, alcohol, and abuse) of 29 A-NHOPI lesbians; 34.5% were totally disclosed to family, co-workers, and health-care providers. They reported high rates of quitting smoking, and low rates of smoking and alcohol

Suzanne L. Dibble, DNSc, RN, is with the School of Nursing; Noriko Sato, MSN, RN, is with the Lesbian Health Research Center; and Ellen Haller, MD, is with the Department of Psychiatry, all at University of California, San Francisco.

Address correspondence to: Suzanne Dibble, Lesbian Health Research Center, University of California, San Francisco, 3333 California St., Suite 340, San Francisco, CA 94118 (E-mail: sue.dibble.ucsf.edu).

The research was supported by Program Grant 4BB 1501 from the California Breast Cancer Research and the Lesbian Health Research Center at University of California, San Francisco.

[Haworth co-indexing entry note]: "Asians and Native Hawaiian or Other Pacific Islanders Midlife Lesbians' Health: A Pilot Study." Dibble, Suzanne L., Noriko Sato, and Ellen Haller. Co-published simultaneously in *Women & Therapy* (The Haworth Press, Inc.) Vol. 30, No. 3/4, 2007, pp. 129-143; and: *Feminist Reflections on Growth and Transformation: Asian American Women in Therapy* (ed: Debra M. Kawahara, and Oliva M. Espín) The Haworth Press, Inc., 2007, pp. 129-143. Single or multiple copies of this article are available for a fee from The Haworth Document Delivery Service [1-800-HAWORTH, 9:00 a.m. - 5:00 p.m. (EST). E-mail address: docdelivery@haworthpress.com].

Available online at http://wt.haworthpress.com

doi:10.1300/J015v30n03_10

abuse. Childhood physical abuse was reported by 34.7% and childhood sexual abuse was reported by 28.6% of these women. Findings from this study will assist therapists with some of the issues affecting A-NHOPI midlife lesbians. doi:10.1300/J015v30n03_10

KEYWORDS. Lesbian, health status, abuse, Asian American, smoking, alcohol, Pacific Islander

A-NHOPI MIDLIFE LESBIANS' HEALTH: A PILOT STUDY

Little is known about lesbian health, especially among Asian American, Native Hawaiian, or other Pacific Islanders (A-NHOPI). These women represent one of the fastest growing populations in the United States. The Asian population is projected to grow 213%, from 10.7 million in 2000 to 33.4 million in 2050; their share of the United States population would double from 3.8% to 8% (Bergman, 2004). One of the broadly defined goals of the 2010 national health objectives is to reduce disparities in health among population groups. However, researchers have seldom targeted this specific population. The health problems of A-NHOPI women are presumed to be minimal since members of this group often do not speak about "private problems"; it is not encouraged in these cultures (Leong & Lau, 2001). Traditionally, women in many Asian cultures handle problems by being accommodating in the situation rather than by being assertive (Yi, 1996).

Population-based studies in the United States have revealed that 4.4% to 11.1% of women report same gender attraction, 4.5% have had some gender sexual activity since puberty, and 1.4% identify as lesbians (Laumann, Paik, & Rosen, 1999; Sell, Well, & Wypij, 1995). Assuming a 1.4% prevalence of lesbians among 150,393,897 American women (US Census Bureau, 2005), there are at least 2 million lesbians in the United States today. The Institute of Medicine (IOM) reported that there are specific health-care concerns that set lesbians apart from their counterparts (Solarz, 1999). These concerns are worthy research priorities (O'Hanlan, Dibble, Hagan, & Davids, 2004). Being a woman of racial/ethnic minority while also being a lesbian is associated with increased health risks (Mays, Yancey, Cochran, Weber, & Fielding, 2002). Lesbians are often stressed by the stigma and discrimination from society and the difficulties of coming out to families. Both acknowledgment and acceptance as lesbians are difficult within their communities and culture. A majority of A-NHOPI lesbians have faced prejudice and have experienced discrimination from being both A-NHOPI and lesbian (Chao, 2001; Lee, 2000).

Previous studies have reported that lesbians tend to have riskier health behaviors when compared with heterosexual women (Bradford, Ryan, & Rothblum, 1994; Bybee, 1990; McKirnan & Peterson, 1989; Moss & Parsons, 1985; Schoenborn & Marano, 1988; Skinner, 1992). These risky behaviors include smoking and increased use of alcohol. In addition, lesbians have been reported to have a greater body mass index (BMI) than that of the national average for women (Koh, 2000; Roberts, Dibble, Scanlon, Paul, & Davids, 1998; Rothblum & Factor, 2001; Valanis et al., 2000). Data from the Women's Health Initiative (WHI) study also suggest that there may be dietary differences between lesbian and heterosexual women that would place lesbians at higher risk for cardiovascular disease and some cancers (Valanis et al.). One limitation of these previous studies was inadequate numbers of women of color in their samples; documentation about the health status of Asian-American lesbians has been especially lacking (Yi, 1996).

The way in which cultural beliefs and norms influence human behaviors is one of the primary issues in changing the risk for disease and disability. A previous national study of lesbians (Bradford et al., 1994) reported that more than half of the sample had had thoughts of suicide, 18% had attempted suicide, 37% had been physically abused as a child or an adult, 32% had been raped or sexually attacked, and 19% had been in an incestual relationship while growing up. Depression and psychiatric morbidity are more common for lesbians (O'Hanlan et al., 2004).

Lesbians who do not hide their homosexuality report more satisfaction in their relationships, although disclosure ("coming out") can result in either greater acceptance and/or becoming a target for violence (Herek, 1991; Tomsen & Mason, 2001). Lesbians' coming-out process is different in every race/ethnicity and is influenced by each individual's community and family support system (Rothblum & Factor, 2001). Asian cultures consider sex as private, rather than a public issue (Chan, 1993). A-NHOPI lesbians fear social rejection of their homosexuality, and they are likely to come out to their siblings two years before coming out to their parents (Chan; Morris & Rothblum, 1999). A-NHOPI lesbians often feel more comfortable in the lesbian community. They have been found to identify more strongly with the lesbian aspect of their identity and are more likely to be involved in social and political activities in the lesbian community than in the A-NHOPI communities (Chan, 1989).

A great deal of medical and psychiatric literature has focused on the issues of women in their midlife years. However, few studies focus upon A-NHOPI women, and almost no studies identify the participants by sexual orientation. Thus, the purpose of this pilot study was to explore the health issues of midlife A-NHOPI lesbians.

METHOD

Design and Sample

The study was a secondary analysis of data collected via a cross-sectional, mail-back, anonymous survey of self-identified lesbians. An adaptive sampling design with multiple data collection strategies was used in the larger study (See Dibble, Roberts, & Nussey, 2004 for more details about the methodology). At the present time, this methodology is the most viable strategy for studying this stigmatized group because population-based methods generate extremely small sample sizes. The surveys were distributed to English-speaking women who identified themselves as lesbians, ages 40 and older throughout the state of California between 1999 and 2002. Only women who wanted to assist with the project were given or mailed the questionnaire packet, and only those ($n = 29$) who identified their heritage as Asian, Native Hawaiian, or other Pacific Islander (A-NHOPI) are included in this report. Because of the multiple distribution techniques used, it is unclear how many survey packets reached an eligible participant. Therefore, the calculation of a realistic response rate was problematic.

Instruments

The 90-item survey form was created, pilot tested, and revised before being utilized in this study. Content validity was established by a multidisciplinary panel of experts. Many of the items have been successfully used in previous studies. Most of the items were demographic in nature such as: age, sexual orientation, education, income, living situation, geographic location, menopausal status, weight, height, BMI, smoking, alcohol usage, and experience with abuse. We examined data in order to describe actual and potential health issues of A-NHOPI lesbians.

Procedures and Analyses

By completing the surveys, the participants indicated consent. To protect the privacy of the participants, the surveys were self-administered and anonymous. The Institutional Review Board reviewed and approved this method of working with this stigmatized group. Besides the original survey, the packets included a postage-paid envelope for ease in returning the survey.

The SPSS statistical software package (Version 13, 2004) was used for data analysis. Data were double entered into SPSS and discrepancies between the files resolved to ensure accuracy of the data entered. Descriptive statistics were generated related to sample characteristics and other variables of interest. Since this was a pilot study, a significance level of .05 was chosen.

RESULTS

Demographic Characteristics

The typical respondent was in midlife (M = 47.5, SD = 7.5, Range 40-77 years), college educated (M = 16.6, SD = 2.6, Range = 12-22 years), partnered (53.6%), and all were residents of California. Most (51.7%) of the women reported that they were of mixed heritage; 27.6% reported that they had Chinese heritage; 13.8% reported that their families were from the Philippines; and 6.9% reported that their families were from other Pacific Islands. Two major groups were represented with 37.9% identified as having at least some Chinese heritage and another 37.9% identified as having at least some Filipina heritage when those of mixed heritage were added to the original groupings. Most of these women were employed full-time (62.1%), lived in urban areas (69%), had health insurance (93.1%), and lived with at least one other person (65.5%). Pregnancy had been experienced by 27.6% of the women and five women (17.2%) reported having an abortion. Fifty-five percent of the sample reported that they were pre-menopausal. Only seven women (24.1%) did not have United States citizenship at birth.

Body Composition

Most lesbians in this sample (57.1%) were in the healthy range (18.5-24.9 kg/m^2) for their BMI; 32.2% were overweight (25-29.9 kg/m^2); and three women (10.7%) were obese with only one of these women being morbidly obese (BMI = 51.75 kg/m^2). These three women were all of mixed heritage. All participants measured their waist and hip circumferences with a disposable tape included in their study packet. The average waist size was 33.6 inches (SD = 5.1; Range = 27-53); hip size was 40 inches (SD = 5.2; Range = 33.5-62); and their waist to hip ratio (WHR) was 0.84 (SD = 0.07; Range = 0.75-1.05). Only 28.6% of these women had a waist to hip ratio in the healthy range of < 0.80. Most women (71.4%) reported exercising at least weekly with all but one of these women walking for exercise. Eighty percent of the exercisers (n = 16) worked out two or more times per week.

Self-Disclosure as a Lesbian ("Outness")

Most of the lesbians in this sample (78.6%) had disclosed their sexual orientation (were "out") to all of their family members; however, 21.4% (n = 6) reported that not all of their family members knew about their orientation. A smaller percentage (44.4%) were totally "out" at their work, most (51.9%) had disclosed only to some coworkers, and one woman was totally "closeted." Most (69%) of the women were open with their health-care providers about their orientation, but some were certain that their provider did not know. Only 34.5% of the women were totally disclosed to family, coworkers, and their health-care providers.

Smoking

Only two women (7.4%) reported that they were current smokers–one smoking 1/2 pack per day and one smoking 1/3 of a pack per day–and had been doing so for approximately 14 years. Many (48.1%) of the lesbians had never smoked cigarettes and others (44.4%) had quit smoking. The average time without cigarettes was 10.0 years (SD = 8.7; Range = 0.5-28 years) and the average length of time that the women smoked was 11.5 years (SD = 8.0; Range = 2-24 years). Three women reported that they lived with a smoker and none of these women was a current smoker (2 quit and 1 never smoked).

Alcohol

Three women (11.1%) reported that they had had problems in the past with alcohol abuse; none of these women were current drinkers. Three other subjects also reported no current use of alcohol. Only two women reported daily use of alcohol, and they reported having one or two drinks each day. More women reported that they drank alcohol only a couple of times a year (29.6%) or a couple of times a month (29.6%).

Abuse

Ten lesbians (34.7%) reported histories of childhood sexual abuse, primarily (50%) by male relatives. Eight lesbians (28.6%) reported being physically abused as children, primarily (75%) by female relatives. Fewer lesbians reported sexual abuse as adults (n = 5; 17.9%) with the major perpetrators being male strangers (60%). Fewer subjects stated they had been physically abused as adults (n = 6; 21.4%). See Table 1 for more details about the abusers.

DISCUSSION

This is the first study to report the body composition, including waist to hip ratio (WHR), for A-NHOPI lesbians. It has previously been reported that lesbians are taller and heavier than heterosexual women

TABLE 1. Characteristics of the Perpetrators of Abuse Against Lesbians

Abuser*	Childhood Sexual Abuse (n = 10)	Childhood Physical Abuse (n = 8)	Adult Sexual Abuse (n = 5)	Adult Physical Abuse (n = 6)
Male Relative	5 (50%)	5 (62.5%)	1 (20%)	1 (16.7%)
Male Neighbor	2 (20%)	1 (14.3%)	1 (10%)	0
Male Stranger	4 (40%)	2 (28.6%)	3 (60%)	2 (33.3%)
Female Relative	0	6 (75%)	0	1 (16.7%)
Female Neighbor	1 (10%)	0	0	0
Female Stranger	0	1 (14.3%)	0	0
Other	1 (10%)	0	2 (40%)	3 (50%)

* Categories are not mutually exclusive

(Bogaert, 1998), and that lesbians have a greater BMI than that of the national average for women (Koh, 2000; Roberts et al., 1998; Valanis et al., 2000). A higher BMI and WHR are independent risk factors for coronary heart disease among women (Janssen, Katzmarzyk, & Ross, 2002; National Heart, Lung, and Blood Institute, 1998; Wilson, D'Agostino, Sullivan, Parise, & Kannel, 2002). In fact, a recent study revealed that BMI had no significant predictive relationship to myocardial infarction (MI) among Asians (Yusuf, Hawken, & Ôunpuu, 2005). In our study, more than half of the A-NHOPI lesbians were in the healthy range (18.5-24.9 kg/m^2) with 10% of the sample in the obese category. However, the risk of developing a chronic illness increases among Asian women at lower BMIs than for Caucasians (Asian Food Information Centre, 2004). Worldwide the best predictor of MI risk was increasing waist to hip ratios (Yusuf et al., 2005); thus, our finding of waist to hip ratios of greater than 0.80 for these women is concerning. Indeed, the Working Group on Obesity in China has recommended that the threshold of abdominal obesity be reduced from a waist size of 88 cm (34.3 inches) to 80 cm (31.2 inches) for Chinese women (Bei-Fan & The Cooperative Meta-Analysis Group of Working Group on Obesity in China, 2002). For therapists, it is important to note that A-NHOPI lesbians who are worried about their weight should be encouraged to do what they can to reduce their waist size and thus their WHR. In addition, therapists should consider the possibility that some overweight lesbians may face additional stigma because of societal discrimination against obese individuals.

Our finding that only 34.5% of the A-NHOPI lesbians were totally disclosed to family, coworkers, and their health-care provider was somewhat surprising. The process of lesbian outness is associated with years of self-identification as lesbian, active lesbian community involvement, and less psychological distress (Morris, Waldo, & Rothblum, 2001). Fifteen years ago, Chan (1989) reported that only 26% of their sample had disclosed to their parents, whereas in our study, 78.6% had disclosed to their entire family. Thus, the low disclosure was more a function of their relationships with those outside the family–coworkers and health-care providers. Substandard care can result from the lack of sexual orientation disclosure to health-care providers, including therapists. Therapists need to create a welcoming environment such that lesbians will feel comfortable disclosing their orientation. For example, registration forms should be inclusive by listing "partnered" as one of the options for marital status. Often, a "don't ask, don't tell" dynamic can be set up if a therapist makes an early assumption of heterosexuality with new patients. If a therapist simply asks of all clients, as part of the routine history gathering, if they identify as straight, lesbian, or bisexual, non-heterosexual women will feel welcomed and more at ease than if they have to initiate coming out to their clinician.

Previous investigators have reported that lesbians tend to have riskier health behaviors when compared with heterosexual women. These risky behaviors include increased incidence of smoking and heavy use of alcohol (Bradford et al., 1994; Bybee, 1990; McKirnan & Peterson, 1989; Moss & Parsons, 1985; Schoenborn & Marano, 1988; Skinner, 1992). Our data are not consistent with the majority of previously published studies that show cigarette smoking to be higher among lesbians. Our finding of a 7.4% current smoking rate may be a function of the geographic design of the study. The lesbians all lived in California, a state with one of the lowest rates of cigarette smoking in the United States (California Department of Health Services, 2002). Our finding of low smoking rates and high quit rates may also be a function of the higher educational attainment of the sample, since smoking rates are lower among more highly educated women. Additionally, our finding of low smoking rates for the lesbians might be attributed to the relatively older age of our sample. Other studies reporting on lesbians and smoking had a significantly lower average age (Aaron et al., 2001; Cochran et al., 2001; Koh, 2000).

The relatively low frequency of alcohol abuse in this population may be a combination of genetic and cultural factors. Asian Americans have been labeled a "model minority," with high rates of abstention and low rates of heavy alcohol use (Caetano, Clark, & Tam, 1998). Asian American women are much more likely to abstain or consume lesser amounts of alcohol than their male counterparts (Chi, Lubben, & Kitano, 1989; Kitano & Chi, 1989). Substantial differences exist among drinking behaviors of various ethnic subgroups. People vary in their vulnerability to the effects of alcohol, and some of these differences result from genetic variations in the body's ability to metabolize and eliminate alcohol (Yin & Agarwal, 2001). For example, after drinking, many Asian subpopulations experience flushing of the skin, nausea, headache, and other uncomfortable symptoms, resulting in their diminished or nonexistent use of alcohol. Those symptoms result primarily from inactivity of aldehyde dehydrogenase-2 (ALDH2), an enzyme involved in a key step of alcohol metabolism (Agarwal, Harada, & Goedde, 1981). For therapists, it is important to carefully assess an A-NHOPI lesbian who comes to you worried that she has a problem with alcohol abuse and describes the "Asian flushing" phenomena. Both issues (metabolism and alcohol abuse) can exist together, but abuse might be wrongly assumed because of the side effects of the metabolic problem.

In this analysis, the most compelling information for therapists to understand is the level of abuse many of these women have endured. Most Asian cultures are highly collectivistic and patriarchal; therefore, open expressions of sexuality or gender non-conformity, especially among women, are a threat to the integrity of the family (Okazaki, 2002). The scope of childhood sexual abuse in the Asian-American communities is largely unknown given the cultural tendency to keep the abuse a family secret. Our findings confirm Okazaki's assertion that a male relative would be the most likely person to abuse the child sexually. One can speculate that the high incidence of childhood physical abuse by female relatives might be in response to a child's gender non-conformity, but more research needs to be done in order to support this conjecture. The roles of "butch or tomboy" and "femme" are more clearly defined within the A-NHOPI lesbian cultures than in White American lesbians (P. Aguilar, personal communication, March 20, 2006). In addition, there is a strong attitude of blaming the victim; therefore, victims endure suffering in silence rather than speaking up. This psychological distress would suggest increased suicidality among A-NHOPI abuse victims; and in fact, the suicide rates in these cultures are higher than the national average (National Women's Health Information Center, 2003). Thus, therapists need to inquire about a history of abuse in A-NHOPI clients, but also need to be aware that the women may be quite hesitant to disclose this information due to shame, self-blame, or stigma. Developing a strong therapeutic alliance in which the client feels safe is a prerequisite for her being able to successfully work through the consequences of the abuse.

To summarize, psychotherapists may be able to work more successfully with A-NHOPI lesbian clients through knowledge of this study's key points. If a woman has an unhealthy waist to hip ratio, therapy may help her develop a successful plan to reduce her weight size and can also be a place to work through the ramifications of societal stigma against overweight individuals. Knowledge of a client's sexual orientation is crucially important in the therapeutic work; however, this study found that many A-NHOPI lesbians do not disclose to health-care providers. Therapists can facilitate disclosure by changing registration forms and by asking routinely about orientation. Unlike other studies of lesbians which have found increased rates of smoking and of alcohol abuse, this study did not; however, therapists should still inquire routinely about substance use. Societal discrimination and prejudice against lesbians, and the complexities of further stigmatization from their own family and culture still leave A-NHOPI lesbians at risk for riskier health behaviors. Lastly, this study's participants had high rates of both sexual and physical abuse in childhood. Therapists should be open to asking about histories of abuse.

Limitations

This study has a significant number of limitations. First, the sample size was quite small because of the age and geographic restrictions of the larger study; however, our results could be used as pilot data for a more comprehensive study. The next limitation is that participants were not selected through random sampling of the A-NHOPI lesbian population, a method that is considered to be the "gold standard" for descriptive data. At the present time, information about lesbians cannot be easily accessed by conventional survey techniques. In addition, since the larger study required that all subjects live in California, the results of this sub-analysis of the A-NHOPI women may not be applicable to women living elsewhere. An additional limitation was that for convenience and anonymity, body measurements were self-reported rather than measured by an unbiased observer.

In this study, all women with Asian heritage were "lumped" together. More than 70% of Asian Americans are immigrants to the United States from over 20 different countries; they speak more than 100 different languages (National Women's Health Information Center, 2003). Immigrants come from places such as China, India, Japan, Philippines, Korea, Laos, Cambodia, Vietnam, and Thailand and represent more than 60 different ethnicities. Each country has its own culture and tradition. Because of sample size issues, we regarded all participants who identified as A-NHOPI as a single group; therefore, some of the individual cultural variations may have been lost. Considering cultural aspects and backgrounds for the health of women in each Asian subgroup is crucial for fully understanding A-NHOPI lesbians' health issues.

Future Research

Our results should be replicated in a larger study with an even more geographically, ethnically, and socioeconomically diverse group of A-NHOPI lesbians of varying ages. Future studies should attempt to gather body measurements in a more controlled fashion and include measures of attitudes toward body size and shape. A future study should explore the consequences of fear and social disapproval, abuse, depression, and suicidality in all the generations of A-NHOPI lesbians. Both qualitative and quantitative research needs to be completed in order to understand the prevalence and consequences of abuse among A-NHOPI lesbians. In addition, the context surrounding the best process for coming out to one's family needs further study. Using heterosexual sisters as a comparison group could be very useful in a future study of abuse, depression, and specific physical health issues.

REFERENCES

Aaron, D. J., Markovic, N., Danielson, M. E., Honnold, J. A., Janosky, J. E., & Schmidt, N. J. (2001). Behavioral risk factors for disease and preventive health practices among lesbians. *American Journal of Public Health, 91,* 972-975.

Agarwal, D. P., Harada, S., & Goedde, H. W. (1981). Racial differences in biological sensitivity to ethanol: The role of alcohol dehydrogenase and aldehyde dehydrogenase isozymes. *Alcoholism: Clinical and Experimental Research, 5*(1), 1216.

Asian Food Information Centre (2004, July). Healthy weight advice–one size doesn't fit all! *FFA, Issue 21.* Retrieved December 28, 2005, from http://www.afic.org/FFA%20Issue%2021%20Healthy%20Weight%20Advice.htm

Bei-Fan, Z., & the Cooperative Meta-Analysis Group of Working Group on Obesity in China (2002). Predictive values of body mass index and waist circumference for risk factors of certain related diseases in Chinese adults: Study on optimal cut-off points of body mass index and waist circumference in Chinese adults. *Asian Pacific Journal of Clinical Nutrition, 11*(S8), S685-S693.

Bergman, M. (2004). Census bureau projects tripling of Hispanic and Asian populations in 50 years: Non-Hispanic Whites may drop to half of total population. Retrieved December 28, 2005, from http://www.census.gov/Press-Release/www/releases/archives/population/001720.html

Bogaert, A. F. (1998). Physical development and sexual orientation in women: Height, weight, and age of puberty comparisons. *Personality and Individual Differences, 24,* 115-121.

Bradford, J., Ryan, C., & Rothblum, E. D. (1994). National Lesbian Health Care Survey: Implications for mental health care. *Journal of Counseling Clinical Psychology, 62*(2), 228-242.

Bybee, D. (1990). *Michigan Lesbian Health Survey: A report to the Michigan Organization for Human Rights and the Michigan Department of Public Health.* Detroit, MI: Michigan Department of Health and Human Services.

Caetano, R., Clark, C. L., & Tam, T. (1998). Alcohol consumption among racial/ethnic minorities: Theory and research. *Alcohol Health & Research World, 22*(4), 233-238.

California Department of Health Services, Tobacco Control Section (2002). Smoking prevalence among California adults 1984-2001. Retrieved December 28, 2005, from http//www.dhs.ca.gov/tobacco/documents

Chan, C. S. (1989). Issues of identity development among Asian-American lesbians and gay men. *Journal of Counseling & Development, 68*, 16-20.

Chan, C. S. (1993). Issues of identity development among Asian-American lesbians and gay men. In L. D. Garnets & D. C. Kimmel (Eds.), *Psychological perspectives on lesbian and gay male experiences* (pp. 376-387). New York: Columbia University Press.

Chao, J. M. (2001). Self-esteem, and coping strategies of lesbians and heterosexual Asian American women. *Dissertation Abstracts International, 62*(3-B), 1568. (UMI No. 3009215)

Chi, I., Lubben, J. E., & Kitano, H. H. L. (1989). Differences in drinking behavior among three Asian American groups. *Journal of Studies on Alcohol, 50,* 15-23.

Cochran, S. D., Mays, V. M., Bowen, D., Gage, S., Bybee, D., Roberts, S. J., Goldstein, R. S. et al. (2001). Cancer-related risk indicators and preventive screening behaviors among lesbians among bisexual women. *American Journal of Public Health, 91,* 591-597.

Dibble, S. D., Roberts, S. A., & Nussey, B. A. (2004). Comparing breast cancer risk between lesbians and their heterosexual sisters. *Women's Health Issues, 14*, 60-68.

Greene, B. (1994). Lesbian women of color: Triple jeopardy. In L. Comas-Diaz & B. Greene (Eds.), *Women of color: Integrating ethnic and gender identities in psychotherapy* (pp. 389-427). New York: Guilford.

Herek, G. M. (1991). Stigma, prejudice, and violence against lesbians and gay men. In John C. Gonsiorek & James D. Weinrich (Eds.), *Homosexuality: Research implications for public policy* (pp. 60-80). Newbury Park, CA: Sage.

Janssen, I., Katzmarzyk, P. T., & Ross, R. (2002). Body mass index, waist circumference, and health risk: Evidence in support of current National Institutes of Heath guidelines. *Archives of Internal Medicine, 162*, 2074-2079.

Kitano, H. H. L., & Chi, I. (1989). Asian Americans and alcohol: The Chinese, Japanese, Koreans, and Filipinos in Los Angeles. In D. Spiegler, D. Tate, S. Aitken, & C. Christian (Eds.), *Alcohol use among U.S. ethnic minorities: Proceedings of a conference on the epidemiology of alcohol use and abuse among ethnic minority groups, September 1985* (National Institute on Alcohol Abuse and Alcoholism Research No. 89-1435, pp. 373-382). Bethesda, MD: Author.

Koh, A. S. (2000). Use of preventive health behaviors by lesbian and bisexual, and heterosexual women: Questionnaire survey. *Western Journal of Medicine, 172,* 379-384.

Laumann, E. O., Paik, A., & Rosen, R. C. (1999). Sexual dysfunction in the United States: Prevalence and predictors. *Journal of the American Medical Association, 281*, 537-544.

Lee, K. (2000). Impact of family origin, self-construal, and acculturation on disclosure of sexual orientation among White and Asian-American lesbians and gay men. *Dissertation Abstracts International, 60*(10-B), 5228. (UMI No. 9948299)

Leong, F. T. L., & Lau, A. S. L. (2001). Barriers to providing effective mental health services to Asian Americans. *Mental Health Services Research, 3*(4), 201-214.

Mays, V. M., Yancey, A. K., Cochran, S. D., Weber, M., & Fielding, J. E. (2002). Heterogeneity of health disparities among African, Hispanic, and Asian American women: Unrecognized influences of sexual orientation. *American Journal of Public Health, 92*, 632-639.

McKirnan, D. J., & Peterson, P. L. (1989). Alcohol and drug use among homosexual men and women: Epidemiology and population characteristics. *Addictive Behaviors, 14*, 545-553.

Morris, J. F., & Rothblum, E. D. (1999). Who fills out a "lesbian" questionnaire? The interrelationship of sexual orientation, years "out," disclosure of sexual orientation, sexual experience with women, and participation in the lesbian community. *Psychology of Women Quarterly, 23*, 537-557.

Morris, J. F., Waldo, C. R., & Rothblum, E. D. (2001). A model of predictors and outcomes of outness among lesbian and bisexual women. *American Journal of Orthopsychiatry, 71*, 61-71.

Moss, A. J., & Parsons, V. L. (1985). *Current estimates from the National Health Interview Survey* (DHHS Publication No. PHS 86-1538). Washington, DC: National Center for Health Statistics.

National Heart, Lung, and Blood Institute (1998). Clinical guidelines on the identification, evaluation, and treatment of overweight and obesity in adults. Retrieved June, 2004, from http://www.nhlbi.nih.gov/guidelines/obesity

National Women's Health Information Center (2003, May). Health problems in Asian American/Pacific Islander and Native Hawaiian women. Retrieved December 29, 2005, from http://www.4woman.gov/faq/asian_pacific.pdf

O'Hanlan, K. A., Dibble, S. L., Hagan, H. J. J., & Davids, R. (2004). Advocacy for women's health should include lesbian health. *Journal of Women's Health, 13*(2), 227-234.

Okazaki, S. (2002). Influences of culture on Asian American's sexuality. *Journal of Sex Research, 39*, 34-41.

Roberts, S., Dibble, S. L., Scanlon, J. L., Paul, S. M., & Davids, H. R. (1998). Differences in risk factors for breast cancer: Lesbian and heterosexual women. *Journal of the Gay and Lesbian Medical Association, 2*, 93-101.

Rothblum, E. D., & Factor, R. (2001). Lesbians and their sisters as a control group: Demographic and mental health factors. *Psychological Sciences, 12*, 63-69.

Schoenborn, C. A., & Marano, M. (1988). *Current estimates from the National Health Interview Survey* (DHHS Publication No. PHS 1-233). Washington, DC: U.S. Dept. of Health, Education, and Welfare, Public Health Service.

Sell, R. L., Well, J. A., & Wypij, D. (1995). The prevalence of homosexual behavior and attraction in the United States, the United Kingdom and France: Results of national population-based samples. *Archives of Sexual Behavior, 24*, 235-248.

Skinner, W. F. (1992). *Trilogy project: Research in the lesbian and gay community.* Los Angeles: 14th National Lesbian and Gay Health Conference.

Solarz, A. L. (1999). *Lesbian health: Current assessment and directions for the future.* Washington, DC: Institute of Medicine, National Institutes of Health, United States Department of Health and Human Services, National Academy Press.

Theisen, C. (2004). In different cultures, cancer screening presents challenges. *Journal of the National Cancer Institute, 96*, 10-12.

Tomsen, S., & Mason, G. (2001). Engendering homophobia: Violence, sexuality and gender conformity. *Journal of Sociology, 37*(3), 257-273.

U.S. Census Bureau (2005). Population estimates: April 1, 2000 to July 1, 2005. Retrieved December 28, 2005, from http://www.census.gov/population/projections/SummaryTabA3.pdf

Valanis, B. G., Bowen, D. J., Bassford, T., Whitlock, E., Charney, P., & Carter, R. A. (2000). Sexual orientation and health: Comparisons in the women's health initiative samples. *Archives of Family Medicine, 9*, 843-853.

Wilson, P. W. F., D'Agostino, R. B., Sullivan, L., Parise, H., & Kannel, W. B. (2002). Overweight and obesity as determinants of cardiovascular risk: The Framingham experience. *Archives of Internal Medicine, 162*, 1867-1872.

Yi, J. K. (1996). Are Asian/Pacific islander American women represented in women's health research? *Women's Health Issues, 6*, 237-328.

Yin, S. J., & Agarwal, D. P. (2001). Functional polymorphism of alcohol and aldehyde dehydrogenases: Alcohol metabolism, alcoholism, and alcohol-induced organ damage. In D. P. Agarwal & H. K. Seitz (Eds.), *Alcohol in health and disease* (p. 126). New York: Marcel Dekker.

Yusuf, S., Hawken, S., & Ôunpuu, S. (2005). Obesity and the risk of myocardial infarction in 27,000 participants from 52 countries: A case-control study. *The Lancet, 366*, 1640-1649.

doi:10.1300/J015v30n03_10

Eating Disorders in Asian American Women: Integrating Multiculturalism and Feminism

Julia Y. Ting
Wei-Chin Hwang

SUMMARY. This paper discusses factors that contribute to the development of eating disorders in Asian American women. We provide a conceptual framework for understanding how culture interplays with risk factors at societal, familial, and individual levels. Because of the complex interplay of factors associated with the development of eating disorders in Asian American women, treatment efforts should target risk factors along each of the aforementioned domains. Clinical issues in treating Asian American women are discussed and treatment recommendations are provided. doi:10.1300/J015v30n03_11 *[Article copies available for a fee from The Haworth Document Delivery Service: 1-800-HAWORTH. E-mail address: <docdelivery@haworthpress.com> Website: <http://www.HaworthPress.com> © 2007 by The Haworth Press, Inc. All rights reserved.]*

Julia Y. Ting, BS, is a clinical graduate student in the Department of Psychology at University of Utah. Wei-Chin Hwang, PhD, is Assistant Professor of Psychology at University of Utah.

Address correspondence to: Julia Ting, Department of Psychology, University of Utah, 380 S. 1530 E., Room 502, Social Behavioral Science Building, Salt Lake City, UT 84112 (E-mail: julia.ting@psych.utah.edu).

[Haworth co-indexing entry note]: "Eating Disorders in Asian American Women: Integrating Multiculturalism and Feminism." Ting, Julia Y., and Wei-Chin Hwang. Co-published simultaneously in *Women & Therapy* (The Haworth Press, Inc.) Vol. 30, No. 3/4, 2007, pp. 145-160; and: *Feminist Reflections on Growth and Transformation: Asian American Women in Therapy* (ed: Debra M. Kawahara, and Oliva M. Espín) The Haworth Press, Inc., 2007, pp. 145-160. Single or multiple copies of this article are available for a fee from The Haworth Document Delivery Service [1-800-HAWORTH, 9:00 a.m. - 5:00 p.m. (EST). E-mail address: docdelivery@haworthpress.com].

Available online at http://wt.haworthpress.com

doi:10.1300/J015v30n03_11

KEYWORDS. Asian Americans, eating disorders, culture, feminism, acculturation

Over the past few decades, there has been a growing awareness and concern over the increase in prevalence of eating disorders around the world. For example, epidemiological studies have shown an over 72-fold increase in the rates of Anorexia Nervosa since the 1950s (Hoek & van Hoeken, 2003). However, despite the abundance of research available on Western populations, relatively little research has been conducted on eating disorders among Asian and Asian American women. The few studies that do exist indicated that the rates of eating disorders among Asian and Asian American women approximate those of other Americans, but have been sharply increasing (Le Grange, Stone, & Brownell, 1998). The notion that eating disorders are a culturally Western or "White female" phenomenon appears to be changing as the international community is influenced by the West.

In this paper, we review the extant literature on eating disorders in Asian American women. Because few studies have considered the role of culture in the development of eating disorders, we provide a conceptual framework for understanding how cultural and societal issues contribute to the development of eating disorders among Asian American women (see Figure 1). In our model, we argue that the risk for developing an eating disorder is influenced by an interplay of culturally influenced risk factors that fall into three primary domains, including societal, familial, and individual factors. Because of the multifarious etiology of eating disorders, no one risk factor can be held responsible for its development. Cultural influences on each of these domains must be taken into account if we are to improve our understanding and treatment of this disease. Intervention and treatment implications are discussed.

SOCIETAL FACTORS

At a societal level, the pressure to conform to changing societal expectations of beauty is believed to be the primary perpetrator for America's desire to be thin. These changing norms are distributed through popular media images and have lead to a "thinning" of America. Why is America's ideal woman becoming thinner? One popular belief is that the social and economic elite set the trends for beauty, fashion, and de-

FIGURE 1. Tri-Level Etiological Model for Understanding the Development and Treatment of Eating Disorders in Asian American Women

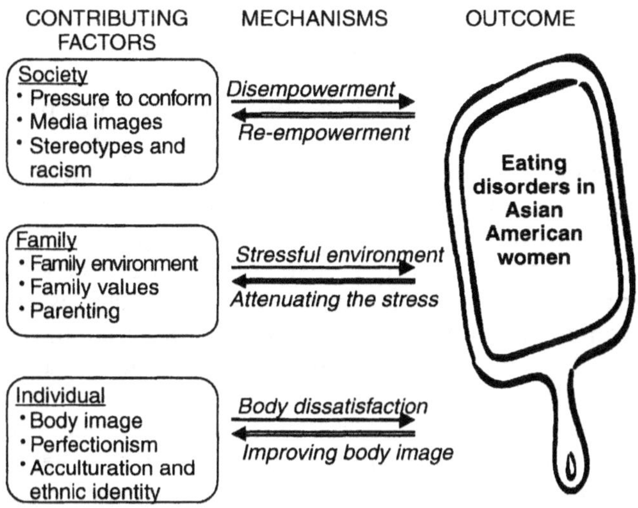

sirability. For example, in conducting the Midtown Manhattan Survey, Stunkard, D'Aquili, Fox, and Filion (1972) found the prevalence of obesity in the highest social class to be one fifth that of the lowest social class. The authors suggested that this continued decrease in body weight among wealthy and beautiful women and the value placed on this ideal thin image by wealthy men has changed America's standards of beauty over time.

As women strive for social, occupational, and economic upward mobility, they may experience increased pressure to conform to the norms, values, and expectations of the dominant society (Mastria, 2002; Root, 1990). This may be especially difficult for ethnic women because they may not fit mainstream ideals and norms (Hall, 1995), and their culture's traditional standards of beauty may also be incongruent with that of the dominant Western image. For Asian and Asian American women, this may become increasingly difficult as they struggle to retain cultural values or meet popular societal images and cultural stereotypes.

Hollywood and media images have commonly depicted Asian women as belonging to one of two categories: (a) the sexy, devious dragon lady and; (b) the beautiful, docile, quiet, and subservient woman

(Chow, 1996; Hall, 1995). These distorted images, which seem to be polar opposites, may lead to conflicted feelings and ultimately disempower Asian women. Moreover, both images perpetuate stereotypical images and may place undue pressure on Asian American women to be unrealistically thin and beautiful. These images are not restricted to the big screen and have, in fact, begun invading magazine ads and college newspapers, where advertisements for diet pills, weight loss, and even eyelid, nose, and breast cosmetic surgeries target Asian American women. These advertisements send Asian American women the message that their ethnically distinctive features do not meet societal definitions of beauty and need to be changed.

Hurtful racial teasing (teasing focused on the target's ethnically distinctive attributes) may further increase the difficulties that Asian American women encounter in their attempt to integrate into the dominant society. Ethnic minority women who have endured racist and oppressive acts often feel a sense of lack of control or helplessness and decreased self-esteem (Fernando, 1984). This, in combination with dissatisfaction with ethnically distinctive features such as being shorter, having single eyelid flaps, smaller breasts, and nose bridges (Hall, 1995; Kaw, 1993), can in turn be a risk factor for eating and body image disturbances.

FAMILIAL FACTORS

A variety of family and parenting factors such as parental bonding and family history of eating disorders have been found to be associated with eating disorders among American women (Strober & Humphrey, 1987; Turner, Rose, & Cooper, 2005). Among Asian American women, parental control and overprotection have also been found to be associated with eating disorders (Furukawa, 1994; McCourt & Waller, 1995). Women growing up in over-controlling family environments through a lack of fostering of independence may develop a sense of inefficacy and loss of control that leads to the development of psychopathology (Parker & Gladstone, 1996). Consequently, these women may develop the cognitively distorted belief that they can re-empower themselves and increase their self-worth by gaining control over their food intake, which is often reinforced by media ads of taking control of one's life through dieting as well as family criticism to lose weight. Kanakis and Thelen (1995) found that eating-disordered daughters perceived their parents as being more controlling and they also felt more pressure from

tions, cognitive-behavioral therapy (CBT) may be particularly effective in treating women with eating disorders.

Perfectionism

One of the main characteristics of people with anorexia is perfectionism. Perfectionistic individuals set unrealistic goals, have selective attention, tend to overgeneralize failure, and evidence greater all-or-none thinking (Hewitt & Flett, 1991). Kiemle, Slade, and Dewey (1987) found that women with perfectionistic tendencies were more likely than nonperfectionistic women to be significantly more dissatisfied with their body.

There is some research indicating that more highly acculturated Asian Americans reported greater perfectionistic tendencies than their less acculturated counterparts (Davis & Katzman, 1999). Root (1990) suggested that this may be a result of the more highly acculturated individuals' attempt to assimilate into the dominant culture and "overcorrect" for any deficits they perceive themselves to have. Perfectionistic Asian American women may be particularly focused on perfecting their appearance because they are ethnically further than other ethnic minorities from the North American ideals of beauty. Failure to achieve an unattainable goal may result in poor self-esteem and an even worse self-image.

Acculturation and Ethnic Identity

In addition to the aforementioned risk factors, level of acculturation also plays an important role in the etiology of eating disorders in Asian American women. Acculturation is a process that involves adopting the characteristics, beliefs, ideals, and values of the host culture (Gowen, Hayward, Killen, Robinson, & Taylor, 1999; Kempa & Thomas, 2000). Root (1990) argued that minority women who identify mainly with their culture of origin may be protected against the development of eating disorders because they are less likely to adopt the North American overvaluing of thinness. However, Gowen and colleagues suggested that increased acculturation may be less of a contributing factor to the development of eating disorders because of world globalization where Asian cultures are increasingly exposed to Western values and ideals before they even move to the U.S. This can be seen when comparing mainland Chinese to Hong Kong Chinese who have received greater exposure to Western culture due to British rule. Lee and Lee (2000) found that women from Hong Kong were more likely to adopt Western standards of beauty ideals than women from mainland China. Compared to their mainland counterparts, women from Hong Kong were slimmer, reported more body dissatisfaction, and exhibited more disordered eating behaviors.

For Asian American women, ethnic identity may further complicate the course of an eating disorder. According to Atkinson, Morten, and Sue (1998), an individual's stage of ethnic identity impacts how they perceive and relate to the larger society. For example, an individual in the Conformity stage of identity development may reject their own culture completely in an attempt to fully embrace the dominant culture. Unchangeable characteristics, such as ethnically defining body features, may be particularly distressing for individuals at this stage and place them at greater risk for rejecting their ethnic selves, devaluing their ethnically distinctive body characteristics, and developing a negative self-image that places them at greater risk for developing eating disorders.

ADDITIONAL CLINICAL ISSUES

Treatment Underutilization by Asian Americans

In general, Asians and less acculturated Asian Americans are less likely than Caucasian Americans to seek treatment for mental health problems (Kim & Omizo, 2003). A number of difficulties including linguistic challenges, stigma and shame associated with mental health services, and less awareness of treatment options may be partially responsible for low help-seeking practices. Because eating disorders have traditionally been seen as a Western culture-bound disorder, Asians and Asian Americans are less likely to seek treatment because they may not be aware of the signs and symptoms of eating disorders.

Under-Diagnosis by Clinicians

Because Asians are often stereotyped to be the well-adjusted "model minorities" and because Asian women are typically more petite than Caucasian American women, mental health care providers may be less likely to assess for an eating disorder in this group. Ethnic minority women have been found to be disproportionately under-diagnosed and misdiagnosed for not having an eating disorder (Thompson, 1994). As a result, symptoms tend to worsen before they are able to receive the help they need (Pike & Walsh, 1996). In addition, Asian-American women may express their eating disorder symptoms as other, more culturally acceptable somatic symptoms, such as indigestion and stomachaches, leading to further misdiagnoses (Yoshimura, 1995).

Current instruments being used to diagnose eating disorders may not be suitable for use with the Asian American population. In a sample of 257 Asian American women, Tsai and Gray (2000) found that an unrealistically low number (e.g., 2 out of 257 [0.78%]) of Asian American women met full criteria for bulimia nervosa. However, if only three of the four criteria for bulimia nervosa as outlined in DSM-IV (1994) were used, the prevalence rate jumps to 5.10% in this sample. This suggests that the DSM criteria may be too stringent when used to diagnose eating disorders in Asian American women. Because of cultural differences in expression of distress, clinicians may need to adjust diagnostic and treatment practices to address the needs of women who meet subsyndromal levels of diagnoses, but evidence high levels of dysfunction.

RECOMMENDATIONS

Based on the literature review and the conceptual framework we developed to increase our understanding of the development of eating disorders among Asian American women, we make the following recommendations to address the issues raised above at the societal, familial, and individual levels. However, these recommendations should be considered in relation to the cultural context of the client and her own belief system. The clinician must use his/her own clinical judgment in determining the appropriateness of each recommendation for his/her particular client.

Recommendation 1. We must re-empower Asian American women through public education, promotion of ethnically-sensitive media images, and the reduction of hurtful stereotypes. Because much of the pressure to be thin stems from societal expectations on women, it is essential that efforts to prevent eating disorders involve public education and reduction of societal pressures. The media should portray women of all ethnic backgrounds with more realistic body shapes and sizes. In addition, the beauty of women from all ethnic and racial backgrounds should be appreciated, not just the stereotypical tall and slim Caucasian woman.

Recommendation 2. Asian American women may be able to regain autonomy and personal control by increasing their understanding of cultural differences in family interaction styles and by undergoing family therapy to correct maladaptive family processes. In addition to other approaches in the treatment of eating disorders, family therapy may be a beneficial form of treatment for Asian Americans with eating disorders. Familial influences play an important role in contributing to the development of eating disorders. Given the importance and stronger emphasis of family and social relations in more collectivistic Asian cultures, creating a supportive family environment for Asian women with eating disorders may be particularly helpful. Understanding the Asian family system, the more traditional hierarchical social roles, rules, and communication patterns, will help the clinician be more effective when working with the family.

Clinicians should understand how the acculturative mismatch between Asian American children and their parents may influence family processes and the onset and maintenance of an eating disorder. This mismatch may lead to acculturative differences in communication and understanding of love and affection. For example, less acculturated parents may express affection in more traditionally Asian ways such as being more critical or using guilt-induction techniques in order to promote behavioral change. Because less acculturated children are exposed to the more physically and emotionally affectionate communication patterns of the dominant culture, they may negatively misinterpret their parents' behavior and conclude that their parents do not love them. Similarly, Asian American children who are scolded about their weight may overinterpret their parents' criticism and develop extreme diets in order to please their parents. The clinician can help the family by helping the child understand that his/her parents did not mean for him/her to develop unhealthy eating patterns. In addition, use of criticism is culturally normative in Asian cultures and used to promote behavioral change, as well as convey love and caring. The clinician should also help parents understand that because their children were raised in the U.S., this method of communication can have a negative and lasting impact on their child. The family and the clinician can then work together to develop new methods of expressing love and affection that can be more effective and benefit all family members.

Recommendation 3. Assessment and treatment of eating disorders in Asian American women should consider both global and specific body dissatisfaction. Clinicians should be specific in their assessment of a client's level of body dissatisfaction and focus on dissatisfaction with specific body parts in addition to global or overall body dissatisfaction. As discussed above, Asian American women tend to show greater dissatisfaction with their ethnically distinct body features than their Caucasian counterparts (Koff et al., 2001). By assessing for global and specific body dissatisfaction and the reasons for such dissatisfaction, the clinician will gain a more complete understanding of the client's actual level of body dissatisfaction and how much of it is ethnically or racially influenced. Treatment methods could then be tailored to address these issues. Clinicians may work with the client to help accept her ethnically distinctive body features. Alternatively, the clinician may help the client focus on positive aspects of her overall appearance, rather than focusing only on parts she is dissatisfied with.

One effective method to address the client's bodily dissatisfaction is to use CBT to challenge the client's beliefs about her body. CBT is based on the idea that thoughts, moods, and behaviors are interrelated. Thus, a change in one domain in this relationship would result in corresponding changes in the remaining two domains. An Asian American client may be depressed about her appearance because she believes that her ethnically distinctive features prevent her from being considered attractive by others. As a result, she may focus her efforts on achieving an attractive and thin figure by controlling her eating habits. A clinician may use reality testing techniques such as referring to Asian American women featured in popular fashion magazines to challenge the client's beliefs that ethnically distinctive features cannot be considered attractive. The therapist can also help the client understand that beauty is relative and culturally influenced and defined. Western standards of beauty are not necessarily the best or the only ideal that people should aspire towards. Working with clients to identify ethnic role models and the positive aspects of their culture will ultimately help empower the client.

Recommendation 4. Clinicians should assess and address culturally-reinforced perfectionistic tendencies. Clinicians should challenge the validity of unrealistic goals set by clients and help clients develop greater appreciation for their ethnic selves. Perfectionistic tendencies and the need to overly assimilate to the dominant culture may be a result of ethnic identity conflicts the client may be experiencing. This, in combination with greater cultural pressures to match up to the "model minority" stereotype, whether academically or socially, can be particularly damaging. Clients may benefit from increased understanding of their ethnic selves and ethnic identity, and their relation to eating disorder development.

Recommendation 5. We must use culturally sensitive therapies that take into account a person's ethnic identity and ethnically-related body satisfaction when treating less-acculturated Asian American women with eating disorders. CBT has been shown to be an effective treatment for eating disorders in the general population (Garner, Vitousek, & Pike, 1997; Williamson & Netemeyer, 2000). However, it may need to be culturally adapted so that it is more culturally congruent with the belief systems and practices of Asian Americans if we are to better meet their needs (Hwang, 2005; Hwang, Lin, Cheung, & Wood, in press).

This can be done in several ways. For example, because Asian American clients are less likely to have learned about eating disorders or mental health treatments, it would be essential to adapt therapy by providing therapy orientations to clients (Hwang, 2005; Hwang et al., in press). Orienting clients to therapy will likely increase their understanding, familiarity, and satisfaction with therapy and, in turn, decrease the likelihood of premature treatment dropout.

Because many Asian cultures place greater importance on hierarchical relationships, social structure, and respect for authority figures, therapists can gain credibility by presenting themselves as expert authority figures who can help the clients resolve their problems. The practitioner may have to be more proactive than normal, take on solution-focused approaches, provide more direction and advice, and teach skills and practices that provide immediate symptom relief early on. In addition, it may be beneficial to focus on the biomedical aspects of eating disorders, and make explicit links regarding how cognitive and behavioral changes can influence physical and mental health. Using biopsychosocial approaches with clients from cultural backgrounds that heavily stigmatize mental illness may help improve client comfort and decrease stigma and shame. Readers are referred to an article published by Hwang et al. (in press) for further recommendations and an extensive framework for culturally modifying CBT to better meet the needs of Asian American clients.

Recommendation 6. In order to increase awareness and reduce stigma associated with accessing mental health care, public education and outreach programs should be created. These programs (for eating-related as well as other mental health problems) can be readily implemented through community and school organizations such as church groups, young Asian American professional organizations, and ethnic student associations. Organizations can promote healthy behaviors by integrating health and mental health awareness weeks, inviting guest speakers, and running support groups for Asian American women struggling with eating and body image issues.

Because Asian Americans may be more likely to seek help from a medical professional first for psychological problems (Cheung, 1987), mental health practitioners could also collaborate with medical practitioners to identify at-risk individuals and increase patient awareness. Family practitioners may also play an important role in reducing the stigma associated with accessing mental health care by normalizing the experience for the patients. Translated psychoeducational pamphlets and brochures that help demystify eating disorders and mental illness can be easily distributed to both parents and youths in such settings.

Recommendation 7. Culturally sensitive and appropriate assessment and diagnostic methods should be developed. Given the problems with accuracy in detecting eating disorders among Asian Americans, current assessment and diagnostic instruments should not be the only method of diagnosing eating disorders among Asian Americans. There is some evidence to suggest that Asian Americans display a narrower range of eating disorder symptoms (Tsai & Gray, 2000), and it is unclear whether those who do not meet criteria evidence similar levels of functional disability as those who do meet full criteria. Current assessment tools should be modified or new tools should be developed that take these differences into account.

CONCLUSIONS

Recent increases in the rate of eating disorders among Asian and Asian American women are a cause for serious concern. This trend suggests that Western influences have penetrated Asian societies and may potentially place Asian and Asian Americans at higher risk for adopting Western standards of beauty and lead to higher rates of eating-related disorders. The changing rate of eating disorders among Asian American women in the past several decades underscores the importance of improving the assessment and treatment practices for this understudied group. In doing so, mental health providers need to consider societal, familial, and individual factors that may place Asian American women at risk for developing an eating disorder. Culture may affect the interpretation and contextual meaning of traditional risk factors such as a higher BMI, parenting styles, perfectionism, and low self-esteem, but may also introduce new culture-specific risk factors such as ethnic identity issues, acculturative mismatch between children and their parents, and hurtful stereotypes and teasing of Asian American women. There is currently a limited body of research available on the assessment and treatment of eating disorders in Asian Americans.

REFERENCES

Atkinson, D. R., Morten, G., & Sue, D. W. (Eds.) (1998). *Counseling American minorities* (5th ed.). New York: McGraw-Hill.

Cheung, F. M. (1987). Conceptualization of psychiatric illness and help-seeking behavior among Chinese. *Culture, Medicine and Psychiatry, 11*, 97-106.

Chow, E. N. L. (1996). The development of feminist consciousness among Asian American women. In D. Y. Wilkinson & E. N. L. Chow (Eds.), *Race, class, & gender: Common bonds, different voices* (pp. 251-264). Thousand Oaks, CA: Sage.

Davis, C., & Katzman, M. A. (1999). Perfection as acculturation: Psychological correlates of eating problems in Chinese male and female students living in the United States. *International Journal of Eating Disorders, 25*, 65-70.

Fernando, S. (1984). Racism as a cause for depression. *The International Journal of Social Psychiatry, 30*, 41-49.

Furukawa, T. (1994). Weight changes and eating attitudes of Japanese adolescents under acculturative stresses: A prospective study. *International Journal of Eating Disorders, 15*, 71-79.

Garner, D. M., Vitousek, K. M., & Pike, K. M. (1997). Cognitive-behavioral therapy for anorexia nervosa. In D. Garner & P. E. Garfinkel (Eds.), *Handbook of treatment for eating disorders* (2nd ed., pp. 94-144). New York: Guilford Press.

Gordon, R. A. (1990). *Anorexia and bulimia: Anatomy of a social epidemic*. Cambridge, MA: Basil Blackwell.

Gowen, L., Hayward, C., Killen, J. D., Robinson, T. N., & Taylor, C. (1999). Acculturation and eating disorder symptoms in adolescent girls. *Journal of Research on Adolescence, 9*, 67-83.

Hall, C. C. (1995). Asian eyes: Body image and eating disorders of Asian and Asian American women. *Eating Disorders: The Journal of Treatment and Prevention, 3*, 8-19.

Hewitt, P. L., & Flett, G. L. (1991). Perfectionism in the self and social contexts: Conceptualization, assessment, and association with psychopathology. *Journal of Personality and Social Psychology, 60*, 456-470.

Hoek, H. W., & van Hoeken, D. (2003). Review of the prevalence and incidence of eating disorders. *International Journal of Eating Disorders, 34*, 383-396.

Hwang, W. (2005). *Adapting psychotherapy to better meet the needs of ethnic minorities*. Manuscript submitted for publication.

Hwang, W., Lin, K. M., Cheung, F., & Wood, J. (in press). Cognitive-behavioral therapy with Chinese Americans: Research, theory, and clinical practice. *Cognitive and Behavioral Practice*.

Kanakis, D. M., & Thelen, M. H. (1995). Parental variables associated with bulimia nervosa. *Addictive Behaviors, 20*, 491-500.

Kaw, E. (1993). Medicalization of racial features: Asian American women and cosmetic surgery. *Medical Anthropology Quarterly, 7*, 74-89.

Kempa, M. L., & Thomas, A. J. (2000). Culturally sensitive assessment and treatment of eating disorders. *Eating Disorders: The Journal of Treatment and Prevention, 8*, 17-30.

Kiemle, G., Slade, P. D., & Dewey, M. E. (1987). Factors associated with abnormal eating attitudes and behaviors: Screening individuals at risk of developing an eating disorder. *International Journal of Eating Disorders, 6*, 713-724.

Kim, B. S. K., & Omizo, M. M. (2003). Asian cultural values, attitudes toward seeking professional psychological help, and willingness to see a counselor. *Counseling Psychologist, 31*, 343-361.

Koff, E., Benavage, A., & Wong, B. (2001). Body-image attitudes and psychosocial functioning in Euro-American and Asian-American college women. *Psychological Reports, 88*, 917-928.

Le Grange, D., Stone, A. A., & Brownell, K. D. (1998). Eating disturbances in White and minority female dieters. *International Journal of Eating Disorders, 24*, 395-403.

Lee, S., & Lee, A. M. (2000). Disordered eating in three communities of China: A comparative study of female high school students in Hong Kong, Shenzhen, and rural Hunan. *International Journal of Eating Disorders, 27*, 317-327.

Mastria, M. R. (2002). Ethnicity and eating disorders. *Psychoanalysis and Psychotherapy, 19*, 59-77.

McCourt, J., & Waller, G. (1995). Developmental role of perceived parental control in the eating psychopathology of Asian and Caucasian schoolgirls. *International Journal of Eating Disorders, 17*, 277-282.

Parker, G., & Gladstone, G. (1996). Parental characteristics as influences on adjustment in adulthood. In G. R. Pierce, B. R. Sarason, & I. F. Sarason (Eds.), *Handbook of social support and the family* (pp. 195-218). New York: Plenum Press.

Pike, K. M., & Walsh, T. (1996). Ethnicity and eating disorders: Implications for incidence and treatment. *Psychopharmacology Bulletin, 32*, 265-274.

Rhee, S., Chang, J., & Rhee, J. (2003). Acculturation, communication patterns, and self-esteem among Asian and Caucasian American adolescents. *Adolescence, 38*, 749-768.

Robinson, T. N., Killen, J. D., Litt, I. F., Hammer, L. D., Haydel, K. F., Hayward, C., & Taylor, C. B. (1996). Ethnicity and body dissatisfaction: Are Hispanic and Asian girls at increased risk for eating disorders? *Journal of Adolescent Health, 19*, 384-393.

Root, M. P. P. (1990). Disordered eating in women of color. *Sex Roles, 22*, 525-536.

Strober, M., & Humphrey, L. L. (1987). Familial contributions to the etiology and course of anorexia nervosa and bulimia. *Journal of Consulting and Clinical Psychology, 55*, 654-659.

Stunkard, A. J., D'Aquili, E., Fox, S., & Filion, R. D. (1972). Influence of social class on obesity and thinness in children. *Journal of the American Medical Association, 221*, 579-584.

Thompson, B. W. (1994). *A hunger so wide and so deep: American women speak out on eating problems.* Minneapolis, MN: University of Minnesota Press.

Tsai, G., & Gray, J. (2000). The eating disorders inventory among Asian-American college women. *Journal of Social Psychology, 140*, 527-529.

Turner, H. M., Rose, K. S., & Cooper, M. J. (2005). Parental bonding and eating disorder symptoms in adolescents: The mediating role of core beliefs. *Eating Behaviors, 6*, 113-118.

Williamson, D., & Netemeyer, S. (2000). Cognitive-behavior therapy. In K. Miller & S. Mizes (Eds.), *Comparative treatments for eating disorders* (pp. 61-81). New York: Springer.

Yoshimura, K. (1995). Acculturative and sociocultural influences on the development of eating disorders in Asian-American females. *Eating Disorders: The Journal of Treatment and Prevention, 3*, 216-228.

doi:10.1300/J015v30n03_11

Finding a Voice in *Shakti*: A Therapeutic Approach for Hindu Indian Women

Neha Navsaria
Suni Petersen

SUMMARY. Despite their growing numbers, Asian Indians in the U.S., specifically Indian women, seek mental health services at a lower rate than other populations, but not due to a lesser need. This paper seeks to present an emergent intervention model for working with Hindu Indian

Neha Navsaria, MA, is a graduate student in the Counseling Psychology program at Temple University. Suni Petersen, PhD, is former Assistant Professor of Counseling Psychology, College of Education at Temple University and now is at the California School of Professional Psychology, Sacramento, CA.

Address correspondence to: Neha Navsaria, Department of Counseling Psychology, College of Education, Temple University, Weiss Hall, 1701 North 13th Street, Philadelphia, PA 19118 (E-mail: navsaria@temple.edu).

[Haworth co-indexing entry note]: "Finding a Voice in *Shakti*: A Therapeutic Approach for Hindu Indian Women." Navsaria, Neha, and Suni Petersen. Co-published simultaneously in *Women & Therapy* (The Haworth Press, Inc.) Vol. 30, No. 3/4, 2007, pp. 161-175; and: *Feminist Reflections on Growth and Transformation: Asian American Women in Therapy* (ed: Debra M. Kawahara, and Oliva M. Espín) The Haworth Press, Inc., 2007, pp. 161-175. Single or multiple copies of this article are available for a fee from The Haworth Document Delivery Service [1-800-HAWORTH, 9:00 a.m. - 5:00 p.m. (EST). E-mail address: docdelivery@haworthpress.com].

Available online at http://wt.haworthpress.com

doi:10.1300/J015v30n03_12

immigrant and second-generation women by incorporating components of Hinduism and an understanding of the cultural ideals and gender roles in Indian culture. Cultural values and religious beliefs are explored through descriptions of the roles of women, impact of immigration, and the ethnic-specific constructs of mental illness and spiritual functioning for this population. Special emphasis is placed on the Hindu concept of *Shakti*, spiritual feminine power, explicating the conflict between the dichotomous roles maintained by Indian women living in the U.S. and ways in which Shakti can serve as a construct of change in the therapeutic process. Information for a therapist to apply these principles even when unfamiliar with Hinduism is provided. doi:10.1300/J015v30n03_12

KEYWORDS. Asian-American, Asian-Indian, culture, Hinduism, multicultural counseling, women

According to recent statistics, the Asian Indian population in the U.S. stands at 1.7 million, which represents an astounding 106% increase over the 1990 Census figures, the largest documented growth in the Asian American community (Humes & McKinnon, 2000). The majority of these Indians, approximately 1 million (Hodge, 2004), practice Hinduism, suggesting that Hinduism is the largest Asian religion in the U.S. (Richards & Bergin, 1997). Despite their growing numbers and vulnerabilities, such as immigrant and refugee status, language differences, negative attitudes toward counseling as a coping strategy (Panganamala & Plummer, 1998), and devaluation of individualism (Das & Kemp, 1997), these Indians tend to underuse mental health services (Panganamala & Plummer, 1998; Ramisetty-Mikler, 1993; Sodowsky & Carey, 1988). Specifically, Indian women are at risk as they are confined by more rigid cultural role distinctions (Hodge, 2004) and may be perceived by outsiders as having an "underdeveloped ego," lacking self-reliance and self-direction because of Hinduism's emphasis on selflessness and detachment (Roland, 1996). Furthermore, Asian Indians are underrepresented in mental health research and culturally relevant interventions in the U.S. This is due in part to the tendency to cluster all Asian subgroups under the nominally misleading umbrella term "Asian" (which for most people evoke the prototype of the East Asian Chinese, Korean, and Japanese populations). Due to these grouping patterns, unique factors, such as the impact of particular religions like Hinduism and specific gender roles for Indian women, can be overlooked.

Religion is a source of positive influence and has only recently received attention in research and interventions in mainstream psychology. Little attention has been shown in either research or practice to the role of religion in the mental well-being of Hindu Indians. It has been found that although practicing psychologists believe client religiousness/spirituality to be an important area of functioning, most do not routinely assess the domain or address it in treatment planning (Hathaway, Scott, & Garver, 2004). Tarakeshwar, Pargament, and Mahoney (2003) contend that religious pathways are relevant for the psychological well-being and adjustment of Hindus and assert that researchers and clinicians need to take into account the multidimensional nature of Hindu religious life. This suggests that religion can be a salient resource for Hindus, in particular women, in developing a therapeutic framework for counseling this population.

There has been emerging research on the large Indian immigrant population (Farver, Narang, & Bhadha, 2002; Hastings, 2000; Panganamala & Plummer, 1998; Das & Kemp, 1997; Ibrahim & Ohnishi, 1997; Durvasula & Mylvaganam, 1994; Ramisetty-Mikler, 1993; Sodowsky & Carey, 1987; Sodowsky & Carey, 1988); however, there remains a significant paucity of existing literature on mental health and psychological interventions for Indian women in this population. Therapy is more effective with a client if an approach is used that encompasses her values and contexts (Sue & Sue, 1999). Therapists' credibility with a client can increase if they demonstrate and communicate an understanding of the client's worldview and acknowledge cultural differences between them (Chung & Bemak, 2002a). Therefore, developing a model germane to a Hindu female's religion and culture is imperative as it can improve the therapeutic connection and provide a relevant context for exploration.

The present authors introduce a model inspired from psychological, sociological, and anthropological perspectives. The cultural role of women in Indian society and its impact on their psychological functioning and coping mechanisms will be presented. At the core of the model lies the Hindu concept of *Shakti*, representing feminine power derived from goddesses. A therapist can effectively use this belief to navigate the counseling process for a Hindu Indian female client. Even non-Hindu therapists can join with a Hindu woman client to navigate the use of this intervention. The paper will further incorporate how any therapist would be able to introduce the concept to such a client. Furthermore, this intervention is not only relevant for first generation immigrant Hindu Indian women, but can be applicable to Hindu Indian-American women, as second and third generation Hindus may strongly affirm Hindu traditional values (Hodge, 2004).

CULTURAL MILIEU FOR INDIAN WOMEN

Roles of Women. Indian culture dictates the content of the feminine identity, which is defined by service to family and society, underscoring the roles of wife and mother (Guzder & Krishna, 1991). Beliefs about a woman's calling is referred to as *dharma* which relates to keeping the family honor, being modest, and putting others first (Bottorff et al., 1998). *Karma* provides a sense of justice in that individuals reap the consequences of their unjust or meritorious actions in this life and the next life (Hodge, 2004). Through the beliefs of dharma and karma, both the psychological and physical afflictions of Indian women may be interpreted as shameful or ill omens for the whole family since a woman's well-being is seen as a reflection of family integrity. Subsequently, Indian women are significantly more vulnerable to shame, guilt, and stigma than men, while an Indian male's affliction is perceived as a cause for sorrow rather than shame (Guzder & Krishna, 1991). Indian women are placed in a unique position due to their role in the family and therefore warrant further research relevant to specific therapeutic approaches.

Although differences in acculturation and generation may impact how cultural values are manifested in an Indian woman's functioning, it is important to note that Indian women generally operate from the same core values. It has been suggested that first generation Hindus retain their beliefs in interdependence and family roles, regardless of how long they have lived in the United States (Hodge, 2004). Second generation Indian American women, having been educated in American schools and raised in an American social environment, appear to be more self-directed, assertive, and verbally expressive. At the same time, this generation shows signs of deep internalization of the core values from the experience of growing up in an Indian family (Roland, 1996). These Indian-American offspring display a strong sense of family connection that ostensibly resembles the Western notion of enmeshment.

This presence of components of both individualized and collectivist ideals can engender a considerable amount of confusion and conflict.

Cultural Contexts of Immigration. Immigration status for Indian women is also of concern to Indian women in the U.S. since they may face psychological challenges in the resettlement process. Not only have they undergone forced migration and loss of family, community, and social support networks, but once in the host country, they may be faced with living in a foreign culture and environment with little or no resources or emotional support (Chung & Bemak, 2002b). Another factor contributing to the understanding of the mental health of Hindu Indian women in the U.S. is evidenced by the alarming number of domestic violence cases. Recent research has shown that two in five South Asian women (South Asian refers to women of Indian descent along with those women from neighboring countries of Pakistan and Bangladesh) in the U.S. have experienced physical or sexual intimate partner violence, a rate disproportionately higher than that reported by other racial/ethnic groups in the U.S (Raj, Silverman, & McCleary-Sills, 2005).

Further exacerbating their vulnerabilities, women in a traditional Hindu context are discouraged from divorce, even if they are victimized, and prohibited from remarriage if they are widowed (Guzder & Krishna, 1991). Threats to choke off U.S. citizenship are some of the most common ways Indian women in this country are forced to stay in abusive marriages (Raju, 2004). Federal law does not allow women whose husbands have come to the U.S with a H-1B work visa to work professionally or petition for a green card individually, thereby making it easier for a husband to gain leverage in a relationship. In the case of domestic violence, the U-visa was developed, under the Violence Against Women Act, to address the immigration status of women trapped in violent relationships. To obtain this visa, a woman would need to report the violence to law enforcement and certify that she will be helpful in prosecuting the abuser. Although the U-visa does exist, it is likely that immigrant Indian women would not know that such an option is available, and may still live in fear that they will be deported if found and therefore stay in the abusive relationship.

Cultural Understanding of Illness. Indian women typically view health as an integration of mind, body, and spirit with a greater focus on the physical than the psychological. Such a holistic approach does not discriminate between physically "feeling bad" and emotionally "feeling bad." There is a tendency to attribute bad feelings to physical functioning. Furthermore, Indian women, in an effort to achieve selflessness, may focus their self-reflection on behavior rather than their own emotions. There are two consequences in providing therapy to women using this way of functioning. First, the diagnosis of somatization that is appropriate for a Western-enculturated client would be inappropriate for an Indian woman. Second, the personal construction of distress may appear for Indian women that there is a dissociation from their mental state or inner self. The dissociation can be construed that for Indian women, there is confusion about one's emotions and that there is an inability to describe or identify one's feelings. Rather than interpreting this dynamic as a deficit, the therapist can understand the dissociation as a cultural artifact and find ways to work within the cultural paradigm to assist the client.

Rather than attempt to tease apart the psychological, physical, and spiritual dimensions, the therapist, following the lead of the client, assumes that when a client reports distress, it has an accompanying psychological component and avoids directly pressing the client for psychological symptoms. By asking for specific descriptions of the client's experience, the therapist can ascertain how the psychology of the woman is affected. After a discussion leading to symptom identification within the framework of the client, the therapist can subsequently explore the sources and remedies. The application of psychiatric diagnosis rooted in Westernized ideals and the subsequent treatments can be detrimental to the Indian woman client.

A social anthropological account of South Asian immigrant women in Britain by Fenton (1996) echoes this notion of personal construction of mental illness by illustrating the elaborate language and symbolism through which South Asian women (in particular, women from India and Pakistan) represent and express mental and physical distress. There are no words in Indian dialects that directly translate to "depression" or "guilt." Therefore, in articulating mental states, a core expression for many women in this study translated to phrases such as "thinking in my heart" and "my heart kept falling and falling" and "my sorrow has become my illness." One woman, after her husband left, received news that her sister passed away which "made the illness grow." Another respondent spoke of the benefit of receiving anti-depressants stating, "My heart grew a little stronger."

The results of this study are telling as they indicate that for Indian women, there is indeed a recognition of distress when these women describe mental anguish. However, there is an absence of a focus on an "I" self, revealing the non-universality of the Western languaging of emotional expression (Fenton, 1996). In a Western form of expression, there is a strong tendency to align statements of emotion with the "I" self, using phrases such as "I am sad" or "I feel depressed." Therefore, there is an assumption that the development of an idea of the "self" as an object is one which may be reflected upon, and acted upon (Fenton, 1996). The Western notion of "self as object" is alien to Indian women. To impose such objectification and separation of the self into a traditional Hindu woman would be a repressive tactic that robs the woman of her cultural supports. Centering the self in such a manner and then reflecting upon it requires an individualistic philosophy, which based on the responses in Fenton's study, South Asian women did not display. However, current Western therapeutic practices call for this type of self-reflection and expression, thus rendering therapy an invalid and incongruent experience for many Indian women.

Responses in Fenton's study also indicate that South Asian women interpret mental distress as originating from an external source, such as a dark spirit, that has consumed their mind, heart, or body. In a similar vein, in India it has often been said that the emotional and physical changes that occur for menstruating women are because at that time women have access to the powers of Kali Ma, the Dark Goddess (Noble, 1991). There is a notion that external forces control mental and physical states and an implication that, to heal oneself, the invading force must be removed. Many Western modes of therapy focus on autonomy and taking control of one's illness which clearly contradicts the Indian attributions to an outside force that cannot be controlled. Such a stance requires the client to move outside their frame of reference to connect with the therapist, which is clearly inconsistent with the therapist meeting the client "where she is." In typical Western therapy, the work of bringing together two competing dualities would involve intense self-focus and often a cathartic experience. In the process of externalizing the problem with Indian women, the therapist assists the client in exploring the outside forces that have led to her construals of distress, specifically exploring her emotional field through her cultural experience of spirituality. The externalization process with Indian women would state, "How have external forces or spirits assisted you in work you consider important?" It is possible for the Indian woman client to remain externally focused as the therapist, rather than directing her attention inward, would direct her attention to her behavior, demands, and roles.

Examining Indian Women Through a Religious Lens

Paradigms of Hinduism. Notions of individualism and autonomy that characterize Western and U.S. culture are in direct contrast with Hindu culture and ideals. For most Hindus, there is a great awareness of and respect for human interdependence and interconnectedness, and if an individual's actions weaken the community to which the person belongs, those actions weaken the person as well (Hodge, 2004). Hinduism is also characterized by rituals which have the potential to ease anxiety, defeat loneliness and promote a sense of security (Hodge, 2004). Therapists can encourage clients to tap into these coping strengths by engaging in ritualistic behavior that reinforces more effective, healthy, and implicit messages. Rituals such as *puja* (worship and devotional offerings to god) and religious fasting reinforce and strengthen an individual's relationship with God, serve in cleansing one's spirit, and serve as a more relevant coping mechanism to provide an enhanced purpose in life. A therapist can help a client develop a routine based on existing ritualistic practice incorporating the client's issues and, if applicable, encourage the client to consult a Hindu priest. Hindu meditation has also been linked with positive outcomes (Hodge, 2004). A therapist can encourage a client to engage in meditation while repeating positive messages that can promote resilience. Meditation can also be combined with imagery tasks to allow the therapist to collaborate in understanding the client's imagery and worldview.

Hierarchical Relationships to the Mother Goddess and Source of Shakti. Indian culture also has a marked emphasis on idealization. Hindu and related mythologies of the idealized feminine-maternal have profound social and psychological implications for many Indian women (Guzder & Krishna, 1991). Indians may attribute mythic status to certain elders, gurus, and others in idealizing self-object relationships or may even identify with idealized mythic figures and gods or goddesses (Roland, 1996). An important distinction between Western culture and Indian culture is that this idealization serves not to direct the social and work world, but rather the involvements in self-transformation to becoming a better and more mature person. For a therapist, it is very important to work with Indian women in this context, as it is one in which they can explore self-betterment. One such context is through an exploration of the Hindu Mother Goddess.

Narratives of Hinduism have emphasized a central matriarchal figure reflected in the powerful presences of the Mother Goddess, variously referred to as Devi, Parvati, Durga, or Kali (Erndl, 1993). The Mother Goddess represents the life-giving, procreative power of the universe (Guzder & Krishna, 1991). These deities also serve very specific functions such as curing diseases and helping people in distress (Erndl,

1993). Generally, devotees use two names, Durga Ma and Kali Ma, to distinguish the duality in her nature, gentle protector and fierce warrior.

The Mother Goddess is the embodiment of Shakti. Shakti represents an overwhelming conscious or unconscious feminine primal force (Guzder & Krishna, 1991). The power of this symbolic feminine entity stands in contrast to the Indian social reality where women often remain precariously positioned in patriarchal joint family systems and are, from childhood onwards, devalued compared to their brothers (Guzder & Krishna, 1991). In the state of Orissa in eastern India, Hindu women will claim that because they are female and share the essence of the goddess Devi, they embody Shakti and the ability to transform the undoable into the doable (Menon, 2002). In particular, Hindu women, in describing the power of their Shakti, assert that they alone have the ability to hold their families together, yet at the same time to devastate them completely (Menon, 2002). The power is great in the sense that it embodies outcomes that are polar opposites and places women in a pressured role. The Kali Ma image is also representative of the unconscious mind that is stirred up by emotional cravings of the heart (Chaudhuri, 1957). Therefore, it is assumed that giving in to Kali Ma will lead to individual assertions and wants, devaluing the family system as a whole and, subsequently, making the family suffer.

Overall, the difficult circumstances of Indian women and the cultural contexts which define their identities motivate the present authors to call for progressive change and a realignment of tradition with changing cultural realities. In particular, with Indian-American women, incorporating Shakti into therapy is imperative because Indian-American women face a strong dichotomy of Indian values versus Western values of autonomy and independence. Therapeutic approaches are needed that are contextually grounded in cultural beliefs. Discussing issues of control and power through the lens of Shakti will provide familiarity to the client and a more traditional agent of change, enhancing the therapeutic relationship and connection.

USING SHAKTI TO GUIDE THE THERAPEUTIC PROCESS

The challenge of culture change is to redefine the cultural metaphors, spaces, and ego ideals that shape life and so establish meaning within the new social contexts (Guzder & Krishna, 1991). Menon (2002) applied this redefinition using Shakti by proposing that for women to become powerful, it is necessary to remake their Shakti through more culturally relevant actions. Our interventions rest in this assertion as Shakti can be used as a therapeutic construct for Indian women to create meaningful and satisfying identities to make choices and take action. The notion of Shakti can be integrated into counseling sessions in the context of a vessel of personal transformation. This Shakti is what gives rise to the form and expression of the "dark side," as opposed to the "I" self, which would be a feared and anxiety-provoking path for Indian women.

The dual nature of Shakti can be explored within the context of a woman's life by helping her to determine how her power is being used and how it was determined that she use it in that way. Whereas, using power in support of her individualism might feel selfish, the woman may be able to acknowledge ways in which she is using that power on behalf of her family, making more negative emotional states acceptable within her cultural value system. Once negative emotions become acceptable, and a woman understands she has control over how they are used, she can integrate them as part of her psyche, identifying with the dual nature of Shakti.

The guidelines for our model follow a *diffused ideology* (Abraham, 2000) emphasizing more dispersed values. Therefore, a notion of fighting the patriarchy in Indian society is not the central value that defines the model. Rather, a set of selective values, such as the ability and strength of the woman within various contexts (i.e., with husband, family, career, society) is the focus. A woman can move toward much greater self-appreciation and self-acceptance while retaining her role in the family and understanding the sense of control she has in determining how to fulfill her role, while still maintaining various facets of a familial self (Roland, 1996). For many women, the family is very important and it is not easy to leave or go against it; therefore, a model that supports the individual while simultaneously making the family and society a viable institution is needed. Guidelines are presented as follows:

Eliciting One's Story of Shakti. Core cultural values continue to influence the behavior of all Hindus, whether they are from lower or higher castes (Menon, 2002). Taking a spiritual history may be an appropriate means of understanding the spiritual capabilities and experiences that have developed over time and inform the consumer's spiritual universe (Hodge, 2004). In a Canadian study examining South Asian women's beliefs on cancer (Bottorff et al., 1998), women who considered themselves Westernized often described other women as holding traditional beliefs; however, traditional beliefs were noted as their own stories emerged. Therefore, eliciting a discussion on religion and culture leading to how Shakti is manifest in the life of a particular client will provide the therapist direct access to the core of an Indian client's value system. This discussion is of relevance as Shakti is a concept that may have historical maternal links, transmitted from generation to generation where Shakti is not only derived from a Goddess, but rather from a maternal elder, revealing distinct family patterns. Eliciting stories from a client can also provide a description of rituals that one may perform that provide an Indian woman with a source of Shakti which speak to that individual's coping mechanisms and sources of strength. Therefore, in assessing an Indian woman's familiarity and understanding of Shakti, we can understand the salience of her spiritual assets.

Identify the Conflict of Cultural Values and the Space in Which It Is Operating. The omnipotence of the idealized object and the unthinkable anxieties of maternal destructiveness are both at work within this conflict in space of Shakti (Guzder & Krishna, 1991). For example, in combining a career and motherhood, Indian women face a number of conflicts. Having a career is fundamentally a family endeavor with an Indian woman's ego-ideal for achievement and success related to the family (Roland, 1988). The experiential sense of Indian women is much more of a "we" self that includes others in the extended family, whereas the American self is an individualistic "I" self (Roland, 1988). The notion of displaying a more autonomous self that must show initiative and be assertive is a source of conflict because it goes against the deeply engrained expectations of the extended family taking care of one's various needs (Roland, 1996). Assisting a client in defining her conflict and determining how that conflict is manifested in one's Shakti is important groundwork in using this concept.

The client elaborates on the cultural metaphor as learned and previously interpreted by her. Then the client and therapist together explore the boundaries of the metaphor, stretching it to fit the new situation in which the woman finds herself. This mutual exploration is done with the therapist in a not-knowing position, asking questions that allow the client to teach the therapist, and in doing so, the client begins to reinterpret in ways that reflect her new environment, new struggles at adaptation, and new perspective through her own cultural interpretation of what Shakti means in her new life. This approach can be used effectively by a naïve therapist as the client leads the way.

Making Their Shakti Moral. Borrowing from Menon (2002), for women to become truly potent, they must remake their Shakti to be moral. This is a difficult task, as Indian women can easily fear the Shakti held within as it bears consequences of protecting the family, but holds an equally destructive force for one's family. To begin to confront the spirit of Kali Ma requires acknowledgement of one's unconscious drives and desires and an acceptance of the existence of an "I" self that would go against Indian cultural ideals and thus appear immoral. However, Noble (1991) stated that for women, the willingness to face the dark is the key to their development. For Indian women, cultural factors have programmed her reality; therefore, this experience can seem "ungrounding" (Noble, 1991). She may begin to fear for her mind. The need here is for work that is grounding to help the Indian woman embody the energies that are awakening in her being, and also for a shift in attitude that makes it all right to feel these new feelings (Noble, 1991). This shift can be achieved by developing how one can use Shakti as an external container that holds thoughts and impulses from the "I" self, but does not necessarily define the core of the individual. In this way, a therapist can explore one's Shakti to understand inner conflicts without forcing a client to explore her conflicts from the "I" contexts. The client is actually encouraged to project her negative feelings on Kali Ma, then reevaluates Kali Ma in her life, and is helped to discriminate between those aspects of Kali Ma that can be beneficial in her life and those that are not.

Using an Indirect Approach to Allow One to Embody Shakti. As mentioned earlier, social isolation for recent immigrants like Indian women results in a lack of meaningful relationships. A relationship with the Mother Goddess can engender a greater connection with one's Shakti where one may shift from viewing it as an external entity to an internalized force with increased self-control. To allow one to embody what is held in one's Shakti, a non-directive approach can be beneficial. For example, Indian women can be sensitive to direct discussions about breast cancer as they may be viewed as insults or even as curses (Bottorff et al., 1998). Approaching the issue through a story of another woman or a mythical Goddess can be more effective. In times of distress, to tide over one's difficult times, Hindu women invoke the help of Durga Ma or Kali Ma through tales of their victories (Chaudhuri, 1957). The personality of the divinity offers a very effective solution in dealing with conflicts and distress. It is said that one can willingly confide it over to the personality of the Goddess, standing outside oneself (Chaudhuri, 1957). A process of embodiment can take place where Shakti is the vessel of strength, the instinctual becoming.

The role of the therapist is as an expert, but devoid of paternalism, encouraging empowerment through identification with Shakti. Even a therapist familiar with the Hindu stories would not know those that particularly impacted her client. Therefore, the therapist asks the client to recall stories from the Goddess and her female ancestors. In relaying the stories, she gains a greater metaphoric understanding of how these forces operate. Typically, the therapist would have the client identify how the stories refer to her own situation in order to use them. However, with traditional Indian women, such a strategy requires a level of self-focus inappropriate for the culture. Therefore, the therapist interprets the relationship between the story and the client's situation. Together, then, the woman and the therapist explore how the metaphors fit the specific challenges she is facing.

CONCLUSION

The article serves to provide an exploratory conceptual framework in which to counsel Hindu Indian female individuals. Although this model warrants further assessment, it extends our knowledge of the beliefs of South Asian women and furthers our understanding of how cultural paradigms endure and allow for change. Along with building a therapeutic connection, incorporating religion into therapy reveals the essence of a Hindu individual's value system, decreasing assumptions and miscommunications. Contrary to other beliefs, South Asian women do recognize mental illness, however, the externalizing language in which emotion is expressed reflects their personal construction of mental distress. This expression of mental distress, along with the notion of a more collectivist self, is markedly different from core assumptions maintained in Western models of therapy, highlighting the need for a more culturally competent intervention model for this population. The notion of Shakti can be used as a container in which to explore the "I" self of an Indian woman in an indirect manner. The Shakti concept is an attempt to find a solution to bring harmony between the conflicting conscious and unconscious mind in a more socially accepted outlet.

REFERENCES

Abraham, M. (2000). *Speaking the unspeakable: Marital violence among South Asian immigrants in the United States.* New Brunswick: Rutgers University Press.

Bottorff, J. L., Johnson, J. L., Bhagat, R., Grewal, S., Balneaves, L. G., Clarke, H. et al. (1998). Beliefs related to breast health practices: The perceptions of South Asian women living in Canada. *Social Science & Medicine, 47*(12), 2075-2085.

Chaudhuri, A. K. R. (1957). A psychoanalytic study of the Hindu Mother Goddess (Kali) concept. *American Imago, 13*, 123-146.

Chung, R. C.-Y., & Bemak, F. (2002a). The relationship of culture and empathy in cross-cultural counseling. *Journal of Counseling and Development, 80*(2), 154-159.

Chung, R. C.-Y., & Bemak, F. (2002b). Revisiting the California Southeast Asian mental health needs assessment data: An examination of refugee ethnic and gender differences. *Journal of Counseling and Development, 80*(1), 111-119.

Das, A. K., & Kemp, S. F. (1997). Between two worlds: Counseling South Asian Americans. *Journal of Multicultural Counseling and Development, 25*(1), 23-34.

Durvasula, R. S., & Mylvaganam, G. A. (1994). Mental health of Asian Indians: Relevant issues and community implications. *Journal of Community Psychology, 22*, 97-108.

Erndl, K. M. (1993). *Victory to the mother: The Hindu Goddess of northwest India in myth, ritual, and symbol.* New York: Oxford University Press.

Farver, J. M., Narang, S. K., & Bhadha, B. R. (2002). East meets west: Ethnic identity, acculturation, and conflict in Asian Indian families. *Journal of Family Psychology, 16*(3), 338-350.

Fenton, S. (1996). Culture, relativism and the expression of mental distress: South Asian women in Britain. *Sociology of Health & Illness, 18*(1), 66-85.

Guzder, J., & Krishna, M. (1991). Sita-shakti: Cultural paradigms for Indian women. *Transcultural Psychiatric Research Review, 28*, 257-301.

Hastings, S. O. (2000). Asian Indian "self-suppression" and self-disclosure: Enactment and adaptation of cultural identity. *Journal of Language and Social Psychology, 19*, 85-109.

Hathaway, W. L., Scott, S. Y., & Garver, S. A. (2004). Assessing religious/spiritual functioning: A neglected domain in clinical practice? *Professional Psychology: Research and Practice, 35*(1), 97-104.

Hodge, D. R. (2004). Working with Hindu clients in a spiritually sensitive manner. *Social Work, 49*(1).

Humes, K., & McKinnon, J. (2000). *The Asian and Pacific Islander population in the United States: Population characteristics, March 1999.* Washington, DC: U. S. Department of Commerce, Economic and Statistics Administration, U. S. Census Bureau.

Ibrahim, F. A., & Ohnishi, H. (1997). Asian American identity development: A culture specific model for South Asian Americans. *Journal of Multicultural Counseling & Development, 25*(1), 34-51.

Menon, U. (2002). Making shakti: Controlling (natural) impurity for female (cultural) power. *Ethos, 30*(1/2), 140-157.

Noble, V. (1991). *Shakti woman: Feeling our fire, healing our world–The new female Shamanism.* San Francisco: Harper Collins.

Panganamala, N. R., & Plummer, D. L. (1998). Attitudes toward counseling among Asian Indians in the United States. *Cultural Diversity and Mental Health, 4*(1), 55-63.

Raj, A., Silverman, J. G., & McCleary-Sills, J. (2005). Immigration policies increase South Asian immigrant women's vulnerability to intimate partner violence. *Journal of the American Medical Women's Association, 60*(1), 26-32.

Raju, M. (2004). *Brides from abroad: How immigration laws sanction domestic violence in South Asian American homes.* Retrieved November 19, 2004, from http://www.abcdlady.com/11-2004/art1.php

Ramisetty-Mikler, S. (1993). Asian Indian immigrants in America and sociocultural issues in counseling. *Journal of Multicultural Counseling and Development, 21*, 36-49.

Richards, P. S., & Bergin, A. E. (1997). *A spiritual strategy.* Washington, DC: American Psychological Association.

Roland, A. (1988). *In search of self in India and Japan: Toward a cross-cultural psychology.* Princeton, NJ: Princeton University Press.

Sodowsky G. R., & Carey, J. C. (1987). Asian Indian immigrants in America: Factors related to adjustment. *Journal of Multicultural Counseling and Development, 1*, 129-141.

Sodowsky, G. R., & Carey, J. C. (1988). Relationships between acculturation-related demographics and cultural attitudes of an Asian-Indian immigrant group. *Journal of Multicultural Counseling and Development, 16*, 117-135.

Sue, D. W., & Sue, D. (1999). *Counseling the culturally different: Theory and practice* (pp. 164-183). New York: Wiley & Sons.

Roland, A. (1996). *Cultural pluralism and psychoanalysis: The Asian and North American experience.* New York: Routledge.

Tarakeshwar, N., Pargament, K. I., & Mahoney, A. (2003). Measures of Hindu pathways: Development and preliminary evidence of reliability and validity. *Cultural Diversity and Ethnic Minority Psychology, 9*(4), 316-332.

doi:10.1300/J015v30n03_12

The Double Binds of Our Bodies: Multiculturally-Informed Feminist Therapy Considerations for Body Image and Eating Disorders Among Asian American Women

Kayoko Yokoyama

SUMMARY. In the dominant culture of the United States (U.S.), Asian American women contend with racial and gender-specific stereotypes that relate specifically to the images of the Asian American woman's body. Recent literature on the body image and eating disorders of Asian American women reveals that beyond the issues of body shape, weight, and traditional diagnoses, issues of racism, racially specific parts of the body, and eating disturbance beyond the traditional diagnostic categories may hold significance. A review of the literature and multiculturally-informed feminist therapy approaches to addressing issues of body image

---

Kayoko Yokoyama, PhD, is Assistant Professor of Clinical Psychology at John F. Kennedy University.

Address correspondence to: Kayoko Yokoyama, PhD, Graduate School of Professional Psychology, John F. Kennedy University, 100 Ellinwood Way, Pleasant Hill, CA 94523 (E-mail: kyokoyama@jfku.edu).

The author would like to thank Sukie Magraw, PhD, at John F. Kennedy University, and Sharon Robinson Kurpius, PhD, and Patricia Arredondo, EdD, at Arizona State University for their continued support and encouragement.

[Haworth co-indexing entry note]: "The Double Binds of Our Bodies: Multiculturally-Informed Feminist Therapy Considerations for Body Image and Eating Disorders Among Asian American Women." Yokoyama, Kayoko. Co-published simultaneously in *Women & Therapy* (The Haworth Press, Inc.) Vol. 30, No. 3/4, 2007, pp. 177-192; and: *Feminist Reflections on Growth and Transformation: Asian American Women in Therapy* (ed: Debra M. Kawahara, and Oliva M. Espín) The Haworth Press, Inc., 2007, pp. 177-192. Single or multiple copies of this article are available for a fee from The Haworth Document Delivery Service [1-800-HAWORTH, 9:00 a.m. - 5:00 p.m. (EST). E-mail address: docdelivery@haworthpress.com].

Available online at http://wt.haworthpress.com

doi:10.1300/J015v30n03_13

and eating disorders among Asian American women are presented. doi:10.1300/J015v30n03_13 *[Article copies available for a fee from The Haworth Document Delivery Service: 1-800-HAWORTH. E-mail address: <docdelivery@haworthpress.com> Website: <http://www.HaworthPress.com>*

KEYWORDS. Asian American women, body image, eating disorders, feminist therapy

For Asian American women, like other women of color in the United States, the body is inseparable from the experience of one's gender and race. The inseparability of the body from gender and sexism has been discussed in the literature on body image and eating disorders (Root, 1990, 1995, 2001). These interwoven dimensions of race, gender, and the body can only be understood within sociopolitical contexts such as racism and sexism. In the dominant U.S. culture, Asian American women contend with racial and gender-specific stereotypes ranging from facelessness (Durham, 2001), quiet invisibility (Root, 1995), and model minority to esoteric sexual objectifications such as the lotus blossom (Tien, 2000) or dragon lady (Shah, 1997). Many of these images relate specifically to the Asian American woman's body. The body is bound by the culture of the times, and the restraints of body image and eating disorders can only be understood by examining both the sociopolitical context and the individual struggles associated with the lives of Asian American women. Root (2001) has noted that the "sociocultural basis for incubating eating disorders" (p. 754) and the literature connecting body image and eating disorders within the context of race and racism is a new and emerging area of scholarly interest (i.e., Mintz & Kashubeck, 1999). The following will review the literature and provide multiculturally-informed feminist therapy approaches to address body image and eating disorders among Asian American women.

SOCIOPOLITICAL CONTEXT

To understand body image and eating disorders among Asian American women, it is critical to consider stereotypes that are based on historical and current oppressions such as racism, sexism, classism, immigration legislation, historical wars, and current trends in beauty and fashion. Negative stereotypes must be considered along with the seemingly more benign stereotypes such as the model minority myth that may serve to hide the body image problems of Asian American women. The stereotypes of Asian American women in the dominant U.S. culture include: concubine, prostitute, mail-order bride, Miss Saigon, war bride, exotic geisha, dragon lady, lotus blossom, China doll, and precious pearl (i.e., Espiritu, 1997). The fetishized (Durham, 2001; Espiritu) and exoticized (Root, 1995) portrayals of Asian American women are also represented in the popular media (Marchetti, 1993; Tajima, 1989). When not being sexually objectified, Asian American women are often absent, portrayed not as ordinary individuals (Tajima), or seen as invisible and dehumanized "busy worker bees" (Root). It is on this end of the spectrum that Asian women are seen as obedient, quiet, and powerless (Root, 1990), all of which echo the voicelessness of Asian American women.

Both new technologies and traditional media promulgate racist and misappropriated images of Asian women and culture which contribute to the objectification and potential denigration, devaluation, or oppression of Asian American women. In the U.S., current Asian trends ranging from fusion food to fashion represent a postmodern appropriation that reinforces the message of the exotic Asian culture. In the fashion world, Indian symbols of femininity such as nose rings and mehndi/henna have been represented by White (not Indian) women. Such trends relegate the identity of the Asian Indian woman to that of the faceless other and privileges White women by allowing them to appropriate meaning to Indian symbols of femininity (Durham, 2001).

In Asian countries, the U.S. media dominates the popular media and reflects the hegemony of popular U.S. culture. For example, in Japan feelings of racial inferiority are revealed in comedic acts that poke fun at the denigrated racial features of the Asian body such as short legs, flat nose, flat face, narrow eyes, and dark skin. White models are commonplace on billboards and advertisements in many Asian countries. A common Japanese denigration is the reference to "daikon ashi" or short, stocky legs that resemble a root vegetable rather than the long and slender legs that are revered in the White feminine ideal. In many Asian cultures, lighter skin has traditionally represented higher social class status as darker skin was reflective of lower class status and physical, outdoor labor. The internet further facilitates the saturation of dominant U.S. media influences in other countries. The increasing Westernization of countries such as Japan and Korea is reflected in media portrayals of a

White body ideal that represent a departure from the reality of women in those countries (Lennon, Rudd, Sloan, & Kim, 1999; Mukai, Kambara, & Sasaki, 1998). Rural regions in Thailand also reflect the universality and pervasiveness of the White ideal of beauty (Sharps, Price-Sharps, & Hanson, 2001).

BODY IMAGE AND EATING DISORDERS

Criticism regarding the influence of cultural stereotypes in guiding the research on body image and eating disorders among women of color has been noted and referred to as the "milieu of collusion" that prevents more inclusive research on the nature of eating disorders among women of color (Root, 1990). Stereotypes such as the model minority myth and subjugated voicelessness may be contributing factors to the lack of research on body image and eating disorders among Asian American women. Some researchers have criticized the overemphasis of body image and eating disorders research among White women to the detriment of women of color (Dolan, 1991; Striegel-Moore & Smolak, 1996). Increasingly, researchers have begun to investigate the cross-cultural differences on body image and eating disorders (i.e., Akan & Grilo, 1995). Yet, Asian Americans may be underrepresented among cross-cultural studies on body image compared to other racial groups (Nichter, 2000). Comparative studies pose problems as the White sample may be seen implicitly as the normative standard to which all others are compared. Additionally, comparative studies oftentimes do not consider or do not have the sample sizes to explore the within-group hetereogeneity of Asian American women. Ethnic-specific values about the body and the role of women in Asian American communities may differentially affect the expression of body image and eating disorders among Asian American women.

Contrary to the notion of body image and eating disorders as a "Golden girl's disease," the research literature indicates that Asian American women do have concerns related to body image. In a study by Robinson, Killen, Litt, and Hammer (1996), Asian American girls had higher levels of body dissatisfaction than White American girls, though the dissatisfaction was not based on actual body fat for the Asian American girls. Koff and Benavage (1998) found no significant differences between Asian American and White American women in terms of body image satisfaction and noted that both groups had similar unrealistic cultural values of the idealized woman with a slender build and large breasts. Despite some studies that found that Asian American women had somewhat less concern about weight and body size (Akan & Grilo, 1995; Chen & Swalm, 1998), other studies have found that Asian American women do have significant concerns about weight and body size (Koff & Benavage; Robinson et al.).

The psychological correlates of body image such as shame, teasing, and racism are complex. As Rudd and Lennon (2000) noted, women may try to gain acceptance through attempts to improve their bodies, and psychological and bodily shame may be connected to disempowerment and body image. Shame has been associated in the relationship between women and their bodies (Rodin, Silberstein, & Striegel-Moore, 1985) and recent research has found initial support for the relationship between shame and eating disorders for White British women (Swan & Andrews, 2003). Shame and obligation are strategies to reinforce proprietary behavior and social norms (Vasquez & de las Fuentes, 1999). For Asian American women, the relationship between body image and acceptance/belonging may involve specific mediating cultural factors such as shame and racial teasing. In a study of South Asian American women, racial teasing was related to negative body image and eating disturbance (Iyer & Haslam, 2003).

In terms of eating disorders, researchers have noted that Asian and Asian American women seem to have lower rates of body dissatisfaction based on body shape, weight, and restrictive eating (Chen & Swalm, 1998; Crago & Shisslak, 2003; Nevo, 1985) and lower rates of eating disordered symptomatology (Akan & Grilo, 1995; Tsai, Hoerr, & Song, 1998) compared to White American women. Yet, Sanders and Heiss (1998) found that Asian American women expressed greater eating disordered symptomatology and fear of fat than White American women. In a meta analysis, Wildes, Emery, and Simons (2001) found that White women had higher degrees of clinically relevant eating disordered symptoms than non-White women. Asian American and Asian British women, however, had levels of clinically-relevant eating disturbance that were comparable to or greater than White women (Wildes et al.). Roh Ryu, Lyle, and McCabe (2003) found that among a sample of Korean females, a few women met the criteria for bulimia nervosa and a high number of women regularly engaged in eating disordered behaviors that would be classified as Eating Disorders Not Otherwise Specified (Roh Ryu). While some of these studies reflect an international sample, such studies bring to question the relevance of current Diagnostic and Statistical Manual of Mental Disorders (DSM-IV-TR; American Psychiatric Association, 2000) categories for the detection of subclinical forms of eating disorders or varying manifestations of eating disorders among Asian American women. While Asian American women may exhibit lower rates of body dissatisfaction based body shape and weight, cultural assumptions of past research may have concealed other racially specific factors that may play a role in the development of eating disordered behaviors in Asian American women. For example, researchers have warned against focusing on global body image as this may serve to obscure more complexity associated with specific parts of the body (Koff, Benavage, & Wong, 2001; Mintz & Kashubeck, 1999; Mukai et al., 1998).

Among Asian and Asian American women, researchers have expressed concerns regarding the seemingly elevated levels of body dissatisfaction based on racially specific parts of the body such as the eyes and nose (Kaw, 1993; Marsella, Shizuru, Brennan, & Kameoka, 1981; Mintz & Kashubeck, 1999; Sanders & Heiss, 1998). For Asian American women, body dissatisfaction may be related to the contrast of the Asian body with the White beauty ideals (Iijima Hall, 1995) and eating disorders may be more aligned with racial loathing than with body weight (Root, 1995). The devaluation of the racial features in women of color may lead to a denigration of one's own race and an embrace of White beauty standards in order to gain power and respect (Root, 1990). Skin color has been a standard by which Asian women can gain social mobility much like thinness is a means for White women to gain mobility (Root, 1995). Racially specific parts of the body such as the eyes, nose, skin color, leg length and width, and hair texture may represent departures from the White ideals of beauty (Iijima Hall).

In the first known study that examined the relationship between body image and racially defined parts of the body, Mintz and Kashubeck (1999) demonstrated the importance of racially defined body parts in understanding the complex nature of body image among Asian American women. They found that Asian American women were less likely to diet or binge, but had lower self-esteem and less satisfaction with their arms, breasts, height, eyes, and face compared to White American women. The authors speculated that dissatisfaction with body parts that could not be altered via dieting may be a contributing factor to low self-esteem among the Asian American women. Unlike the White American women in the study, body dissatisfaction did not lead to dieting behaviors among Asian American women (Mintz & Kashubeck). In further support, Koff, Benavage, and Wong (2001) found that Asian American and White American women were similarly dissatisfied with their bodies, but that Asian American women were less satisfied with their stomach, shoulders, arms, face, hair, and height. Kennedy, Templeton, Gandhi, and Gorzalka (2004) found that male and female Chinese Canadians and Indo-Asians were less satisfied with their body image compared to European Canadians, with Chinese Canadians being least satisfied with their facial attractiveness and specific body parts. Chinese Canadian women were the most dissatisfied with their breast size (Kennedy et al.).

The literature reveals that Asian American women exhibit complex and multilayered considerations associated with body image and eating disordered behaviors. Markey (2004) outlined a tripartite model of the cultural development of eating disorders. In this model, the three main influences include eating behaviors, body image ideals, and health perception. The family-specific and cultural socialization of eating and the subjective perception of health and disease need to be further explored as an influence in the development of eating disorders among Asian American women. Further studies are needed to expand the understanding of body image and eating disorders among Asian American women, with particular attention to variations due to ethnicity (Kennedy et al., 2004), social class, sexual orientation (Walcott, Pratt, & Patel, 2003), and preadolescence (Root, 2001).

TREATMENT CONSIDERATIONS

The research on the treatment of eating disorders for women of color is limited (Stein, Saelens, Dounchis, Lewczyk, Swenson, & Wilfley, 2001). The following will address general treatment considerations and then provide perspectives on multiculturally-informed feminist approaches to the treatment of body image and eating disorder issues for Asian American women. Both feminist therapy (i.e., Israeli & Santor, 2000) and the multicultural guidelines endorsed by the American Psychological Association (APA) in 2002 (APA, 2003) emphasize the importance of sociopolitical context. The multicultural guidelines or multicultural counseling competencies (MCCs) are reflective of both culturally and ethically responsive practice, and integrating them into specific clinical issues within specific cultural groups represents the next phase of direction for the multicultural guidelines (Arredondo & Toporek, 2004).

In keeping with the MCCs, a multiculturally competent clinical assessment of body image and eating disorders among Asian American women should first consider the biases, values, and assumptions of the therapist and how these affect the intersubjective meanings created within the therapeutic relationship. Therapists' own awareness of themselves as a racial, cultural, and gendered being will greatly affect the therapeutic relationship. Racial identity, ethnic identity, and acculturation status need to be considered along with gender role traditionality, sexual orientation, spiritual/religious identification, social class, and disability issues. [Readers are referred to Arredondo, Toporek, Brown, Sanchez, Locke, Sanchez et al. (1996) for a review of the Dimensions of Personal Identity model that elucidates a model on complex personal identities.] Clinicians must consider these complex identities within the context of the cultural and family messages directed at the Asian American woman about the body and eating. Additionally, developmental concerns such as adolescence or major life changes such as immigration need to be considered as they often trigger the onset or exacerbate disordered eating or body image problems.

In terms of comorbidity, Wooley (1994) provided evidence for the relationship between sexual abuse and eating disorders and noted the gender politics debate surrounding this issue. Eating disorders may be considered a symptom of trauma and may initially develop as a meaningful and powerful way to cope (Root, 1991). For Asian American women, an eating disorder may be a way to "give voice" to the trauma without bringing shame and saving face for the family. Successful treatment warrants the need to address trauma issues in conjunction with body image or eating disordered problems (Root, 2001), and therapists must pay attention to the relevant clinical, cultural, and sociopolitical issues.

Emphasis should be placed on the need to consider the continuum of distress. Body image and eating disordered behaviors are best understood on a continuum from little or no distress to severe and life-threatening levels of distress, with many women falling in the middle (Thompson, Henberg, Altabe, & Tantleff-Dunn, 1999). The difference between levels of clinically significant distress and what is known as the "normative discontent" (Rodin et al., 1985) is a fine distinction (Thompson et al.). For Asian American women, the need to consider body image and eating disordered behaviors on this continuum is particularly important as studies indicate that there are high numbers of women who do not fit the traditional DSM categories and who exhibit subclinical eating disordered behaviors (Wildes et al., 2001).

The recent literature on body image has focused on the multidimensional aspects of the body image construct (Fisher, 1990). The term "body image" has been used in a variety of contexts with a divergence of meanings. Researchers have reinforced the need for more complex assessment of body image because studies examining specific parts of the body (beyond the surface of global body image or overall appearance) have revealed racial and ethnic differences among women (Miller, Gleaves, Hirsch, Green, Snow, & Corbett., 2000). Koff and Benavage (1998) upheld the notion that women form judgments about their bodies on a part-by-part basis and that these differing parts may have differential effects on body image. Recent studies have indicated that Asian American women exhibit dissatisfaction that may be specific to body parts that depart from the White ideals of beauty (Mintz & Kashubeck, 1999). Racially specific parts of the body, such as the eyes, nose, lips, skin color, hair texture, and leg length, that have not been "traditionally assessed" warrants attention (Root, 2001). Clinicians must maintain awareness of the complexity of body image and explore beyond the boundaries of general appearance, weight, or dieting to consider specific body parts, racial teasing, and subclinical forms of eating disordered behaviors.

FEMINIST APPROACHES TO THERAPY AND PREVENTION

Due to the tremendous diversity among Asian American women, identification with the term "feminist" may differ and for some, feminism may be perceived as reflecting a White and middle-class agenda (Brown, 1995). As Yuri Kochiyama, a prominent Asian American activist, noted, "So much of the White women's movement was about equal pay and upward mobility. They didn't really understand the damage of racism on the human psyche" (Fujino, 1997). Though Asian women in the U.S. have been organizing since the Asian American movement of the 1960s and continue to make strides toward social justice (Shah, 1997), Asian American feminism may be considered to be in its infancy (Chow, 1996) and identification with the term "feminist" may vary. For some Asian American women, values such as obedience and filial piety may moderate the development of a feminist consciousness (Chow, 1987). Given, however, that all Asian American women exist within a dominant U.S. culture that is racist and sexist, feminist approaches to therapy warrant consideration. Feminist therapy may be the primary theoretical orientation or feminist approaches may be integrated into the framework of another theoretical orientation.

Israeli and Santor (2000) reviewed the extant literature on feminist therapy and found that feminist therapy reflects four major core components: consciousness raising; social and gender role analysis; resocialization; and social activism. These four components have been adapted for use with Asian American women in addressing body image and eating disorder issues. Consciousness raising may involve attempts to connect the gendered or racial aspects of the body into a social context with statements such as, "You're really becoming aware of how this society views Asian American women." While all symptoms need to be taken seriously and not all aspects of body image or eating disorders should be externalized, consciousness raising is an opportunity to assess, clarify, and scrutinize the sociopolitical dimensions of the distress. Social and gender role analysis may involve an exploration of the messages from the family of origin about the body. This analysis provides an opportunity to assess relationships and to identify the individual meanings associated with the body as an Asian American woman ("How have your relationships influenced how you feel about your body/race?"). Resocialization provides an opportunity to practice new coping strategies on a cognitive and behavioral level and to redefine previous or traditional role expectations with statements such as, "It seems confusing to know how to balance being respectful to your family and culture while also asserting what you need or know to be true. Yet you've made gains in asserting your needs. What's helped you to do this so far?" Finally, social activism differs in that it involves the integration of political advocacy with therapy. For some Asian American women, being an activist and exposing the oppressions related to being an Asian American woman toward social change may provide significant meaning, purpose, and healing. Given these four components, there may be a wide range of approaches to address these components in actual practice.

Giving voice and exploring power dynamics represent an important first step in addressing body image and eating disorders. Olson (1995) provides an example of collaborative feminist approaches and the use of writing in working with women with eating disorders. In therapy, the therapist and client engage in a shared and collaborative dialogue. Olson asserts that collaborative dialogue gives rise to the client's sense of voice and expression, and aids in "naming" and "restorying" the experience. Through the power to self-define her experience within the connection of the therapeutic relationship, the voice is able to emerge over the body as the expressive vehicle. Through this process, writing represents a strategy to incorporate and facilitate this newly developing sense of self and self-expression (Olson). For Asian American women, writing stands as a potent strategy that encourages communication with self and others in ways that may be culturally consistent as it relies less on more verbal forms of expression valued in traditional forms of therapy. In practice, this author has witnessed significant transformations with the use of writing as a vehicle for voice and empowerment in working with Asian American women with body image and eating disorders.

Faith, Pinhas, Schmelefske, and Bryden (2003) developed a feminist-informed model for joint decision-making in the treatment of eating disorders. In this model, a multidisciplinary team of professionals (including psychiatrists, dieticians, physicians, therapists, family workers, and teachers) practice transparency in communicating treatment options and the client works collaboratively with the staff. To the extent that it may be medically safe, clients are encouraged to raise their concerns, be active in the treatment planning, and practice self-determination toward recovery. One study has found initial support for collaborative interventions in the treatment of eating disorders (Geller, Brown, Zaitsoff, Goodrich, & Hastings, 2003). Such collaborative interventions take into consideration client readiness and motivation for change (Geller et al.). Treatment is noncoercive, supportive, empowering, and educational in regards to consciousness raising, as well as nutritional and physical health. While Asian values around relationship hierarchies may reflect a more formal regard for the "doctor-patient" relationship, a collaborative, family-based approach to decision-making may be one of the culturally relevant strategies built around a more active, client-initiated treatment plan. Reflective practice is a cornerstone of this model wherein the multidisciplinary team considers the clinical and ethical dimensions of the treatment with authentic reflection of the feedback from the clients and families and the impact of secondary trauma on the staff themselves (Faith et al.). Reflective practice can be extended to be consistent with the multicultural guidelines (APA, 2003) by enhancing therapist self-awareness by exploring the biases, assumptions, fears, and values of the therapist and examining the sociopolitical issues of racism and sexism that influence the expression of eating disorders and body image issues among Asian American women.

Finally, the prevention of eating disorders and body image issues among Asian American women is crucial given the large role of sociocultural factors. In recent years, positive psychology has gained prominence in the psychological literature (Seligman & Csikszentmihalyi, 2000), yet has been criticized for its monocultural agenda (D'Andrea, 2005). The principles of positive psychology may be integrated with feminist and multicultural perspectives to address the powerful forces at work in the maintenance of eating disorders and body image issues. Steck, Abrams, and Phelps (2004) reviewed various positive prevention programs and proposed an eating disorders prevention model based on the three pillars of positive psychology (subjective well-being, constructive individual traits, and positive institutions). Subjective well-being and the development of constructive individual traits may be enhanced through prevention programs that emphasize active involvement and psychoeducation toward the development of coping mechanisms such as "active media combat" of inappropriate messages around body ideals. For Asian American women, constructive individual traits such as coping mechanisms and self-esteem may be developed by combating negative media stereotypes and encouraging knowledge around positive Asian American values and role models. Additionally, reframing the positive qualities of one's body, including gender-specific and Asian racial features, may help to combat body dissatisfaction. In terms of positive institutions, the involvement of family and teachers in prevention programs, as well as encouraging positive peer interactions were noted as possible protective factors in the prevention of eating disorders (Steck et al.). Asian American parents may benefit from becoming aware of the importance of body image and eating issues in the success and healthy development of young women. Learning about how eating disordered behaviors may be giving voice to the concerns of these young women may help families address feelings and conflicts in a culturally consistent manner. Psychoeducational and preventative efforts may also serve, in part, to de-stigmatize mental health issues such as body image and eating disorders in the Asian American community.

CONCLUSION

Women are often caught in a double bind in regards to their bodies. For Asian American women, negative stereotypes and messages about the ideal body from the dominant U.S. culture and their culture of origin may conflict with reality, restrict healthy attitudes toward one's body, and result in a particularly toxic situation. Tien (2000) warned that repeated exposure to denigrating images may have a negative effect on the psychosexual identity development of Asian American women, yet there are also injunctions against defining oneself in terms of race, ethnicity, or gender in this melting pot, color-blind dominant U.S. culture. For some Asian American women, stressors such as racism and sexism may manifest in body image and eating disordered behaviors. One way out of the negative spiral of this double bind is to understand and expose both the social and individual foundations that sustain the body image or eating disorder. In this way, the feminist therapist and the Asian American woman join together in a powerful way to voice and explore the many layered meanings associated with the complex issues of body image and eating disorders.

REFERENCES

Akan, G. E., & Grilo, C. M. (1995). Sociocultural influences on eating attitudes and behaviors, body image, and psychosocial functioning: A comparison of African-American, Asian-American, and Caucasian college women. *International Journal of Eating Disorders, 18*(2), 181-187.

American Psychiatric Association (2000). *Diagnostic and statistical manual of mental disorders* (4th ed.). Washington, DC: Author.

American Psychological Association (2003). Guidelines on multicultural education, training, research, practice, and organizational change for psychologists. *American Psychologist, 58*(5), 377-402.

Arredondo, P., & Toporek, R. (2004). Multicultural counseling competencies = Ethical practice. *Journal of Mental Health Counseling, 26*(1), 44-55.

Arredondo, P., Toporek, R., Brown, S. P., Sanchez, J., Locke, D. C., Sanchez, J. et al. (1996). Operationalization of the multicultural counseling competencies. *Journal of Multicultural Counseling and Development, 24*(1), 42-78.

Brown, L. S. (1995). Cultural diversity in feminist therapy: Theory and practice. In H. Landrine (Ed.), *Bringing cultural diversity to feminist psychology* (pp. 143-162). Washington, DC: American Psychological Association.

Chen, W., & Swalm, R. L. (1998). Chinese and American college students' body-image: Perceived body shape and body affect. *Perceptual and Motor Skills, 87*(2), 395-403.

Chow, E. N-L. (1987). The development of a feminist consciousness among Asian American women. *Gender and Society, 1*(3), 284-299.

Chow, E. N-L. (1996). *Race, class, & gender: Common bonds, different voices.* Thousand Oaks, CA: Sage.

Crago, M., & Shisslak, C. M. (2003). Ethnic differences in dieting, binge eating, and purging behaviors among American females: A review. *Eating Disorders, 11*, 289-304.

D'Andrea, M. (2005, January). *Reclaiming positive psychology from a multicultural perspective: Combating new forms of racism and ethnocentrism in psychology.* Presentation at the National Multicultural Conference and Summit, Hollywood, CA.

Dolan, B. (1991). Cross-cultural aspects of anorexia nervosa and bulimia: A review. *International Journal of Eating Disorders, 20*, 67-78.

Durham, M. G. (2001). Displaced persons: Symbols of South Asian femininity and the returned gaze in U.S. media culture. *Communication Theory, 11*(2), 201-217.

Espiritu, Y. L. (1996). *Asian American women and men.* Thousand Oaks, CA: Sage.

Faith, K., Pinhas, L., Schmelefske, J., & Bryden, P. (2003). Developing a feminist-informed model for decision making in the treatment of adolescent eating disorders. *Eating Disorders, 11*, 305-315.

Fisher, S. (1990). The evolution of psychological concepts about the body. In T. F. Cash & Pruzinsky (Eds.), *Body images: Development, deviance, and change* (pp. 3-20). New York: Guilford.

Fujino, D. C. (1997). Revolution from the heart: The making of an Asian American woman activist, Yuri Kochiyama. In S. Shah (Ed.), *Dragon ladies: Asian American feminists breathe fire* (pp. 169-181). Boston: South End Press.

Geller, J., Brown, K. E., Zaitsoff, S. L., Goodrich, S., & Hastings, F. (2003). Collaborative versus directive interventions in the treatment of eating disorders: Implications for care providers. *Professional Psychology: Research and Practice, 34*(4), 406-413.

Iijima Hall, C. C. (1995). Asian eyes: Body image and eating disorders of Asian and Asian American women. *Eating Disorders, 3*(1), 8-19.

Israeli, A. L., & Santor, D. A. (2000). Reviewing effective components of feminist therapy. *Counseling Psychology Quarterly, 13*(3), 233-247.

Iyer, D. S., & Haslam, N. (2003). Body image and eating disturbance among South Asian-American women: The role of racial teasing. *International Journal of Eating Disorders, 34*, 142-147.

Kaw, E. (1993). Medicalization of racial features: Asian American women and cosmetic surgery. *Medical Anthropology Quarterly, 7*(1), 74-89.

Kennedy, M. A., Templeton, L., Gandhi, A., & Gorzalka, B. B. (2004). Asian body image satisfaction: Ethnic and gender differences across Chinese, Indo-Asian, and European-Descent students. *Eating Disorders, 12*, 321-336.

Koff, E., & Benavage, A. (1998). Breast size perception and satisfaction, body image, and psychological functioning in Caucasian and Asian American college women. *Sex Roles, 38*, 655-673.

Koff, E., Benavage, A., & Wong, B. (2001). Body-image attitudes and psychosocial functioning in Euro-American and Asian-American college women. *Psychological Reports, 88*, 917-928.

Lennon, S. J., Rudd, N. A., Sloan, B., & Kim, J. S. (1999). Attitudes toward gender roles, self-esteem, and body image: Application of a model. *Clothing and Textiles Research Journal, 17*(4), 191-202.

Marchetti, G. (1993). *Romance and the "yellow peril": Race, sex, and discursive strategies in Hollywood fiction.* Berkeley, CA: University of California Press.

Markey, C. N. (2004). Culture and the development of eating disorders: A tripartite model. *Eating Disorders, 12*, 139-156.

Marsella, A. J., Shizuru, L., Brennan, J., & Kameoka, V. (1981). Depression and body image satisfaction. *Journal of Cross-Cultural Psychology, 12*, 360-371.

Miller, K. J., Gleaves, D. H., Hirsch, T. G., Green, B. A., Snow, A. C., & Corbett, C. C. (2000). Comparisons of body image dimensions by race/ethnicity and gender in a university population. *International Journal of Eating Disorders, 27*(3), 310-316.

Mintz, L. B., & Kashubeck, S. (1999). Body image and disordered eating among Asian American and Caucasian college students: An examination of race and gender differences. *Psychology of Women Quarterly, 23*(4), 781-796.

Mukai, T., Kambara, A., & Sasaki, Y. (1998). Body dissatisfaction, need for social approval, and eating disturbances among Japanese and American college women. *Sex Roles, 39,* 751-763.

Nevo, S. (1985). Bulimic symptoms: Prevalence and ethnic differences among college women. *International Journal of Eating Disorders, 4,* 151-168.

Nichter, M. (2000). *Fat talk: What girls and their parents say about dieting.* Cambridge, MA: Harvard University Press.

Olson, M. E. (1995). Conversation and writing: A collaborative approach to bulimia. *Journal of Feminist Family Therapy, 6*(4), 21-44.

Robinson, T. N., Killen, J. D., Litt, I. F., & Hammer, L. (1996). Ethnicity and body dissatisfaction: Are Hispanic and Asian girls at increased risk for eating disorders? *Journal of Adolescent Health, 19*(6), 384-393.

Rodin, J., Silberstein, L., & Striegel-Moore, R. (1985). Women and weight: A normative discontent. In T. B. Sonderegger (Ed.), *Nebraska Symposium on Motivation* (vol. 32; pp. 267-307). Lincoln, NE: University of Nebraska Press.

Roh Ryu, H., Lyle, R. M., & McCabe, G. P. (2003). Factors associated with weight concerns and unhealthy eating patterns among young Korean females. *Eating Disorders, 11,* 129-141.

Root, M. P. P. (1990). Disordered eating in women of color. *Sex Roles*, *22*(7/8), 525-536.

Root, M. P. P. (1995). The psychology of Asian American women. In H. Landrine (Ed.), *Bringing cultural diversity to feminist psychology* (pp. 265-302). Washington, DC: American Psychological Association.

Root, M. P. P. (2001). Future considerations in research on eating disorders. *The Counseling Psychologist, 29*(5), 754-762.

Rudd, N. A., & Lennon, S. J. (2000). Body image and appearance management behaviors in college women. *Clothing and Textiles Research Journal, 18*(3), 152-162.

Sanders, N. M., & Heiss, C. J. (1998). Eating attitudes and body image of Asian and Caucasian college women. *Eating Disorders: The Journal of Treatment and Prevention, 6,* 15-27.

Seligman, M. E. P., & Czikszentmihalyi, M. (2000). Positive psychology: An introduction. *American Psychologist, 55,* 5-14.

Shah, S. (1997). Introduction: Slaying the dragon lady. In S. Shah (Ed.), *Dragon ladies: Asian American feminists breathe fire* (pp. xii-xxi). Boston: South End Press.

Sharps, M. J., Price-Sharps, J. L., & Hanson, J. (2001). Body image preference in the United States and rural Thailand: An exploratory study. *The Journal of Psychology, 135*(5), 518-526.

Steck, E. L., Abrams, L. M., & Phelps, L. (2004). Positive psychology in the prevention of eating disorders. *Psychology in the Schools, 41*(1), 111-117.

Stein, R. I., Saelens, B. E., Dounchis, J. Z., Lewczyk, C. M., Swenson, A. K., & Wilfley, D. E. (2001). Treatment of eating disorders in women. *The Counseling Psychologist, 29*(5), 695-732.

Striegel-Moore, R., & Smolak, L. (1996). The role of race in the development of eating disorders. In L. Smolak, M. Levine, & R. Striegel-Moore (Eds.), *The developmental psychopathology of eating disorders* (pp. 259-285). New Jersey: Erlbaum.

Swan, S., & Andrews, B. (2003). The relationship between shame, eating disorders and disclosure in treatment. *British Journal of Clinical Psychology, 42*, 367-378.

Tajima, R. E. (1989). Lotus blossoms don't bleed: Images of Asian women. In Asian Women United of California (Ed.), *Making waves: An anthology of writings by and about Asian American women* (pp. 308-317). Boston: Beacon Press.

Thompson, K. J., Henberg, J. L., Altabe, M., & Tantleff-Dunn, S. (1999). *Exacting beauty: Theory, assessment, and treatment of body image disturbance.* Washington, DC: American Psychological Association.

Tien, L. (2000). U.S. attitudes toward women of Asian ancestry: Legislative and media perspectives. In J. L. Chin (Ed.), *Relationships among Asian American women* (pp. 29-48). Washington, DC: American Psychological Association.

Tsai, C. Y., Hoerr, S. L., & Song, W. O. (1998). Dieting behavior of Asian college women attending a U.S. university. *Journal of American College Health, 46*(4), 163-168.

Vasquez, M. J. T., & de las Fuentes, C. (1999). American-born Asian, African, Latina, and American Indian adolescent girls: Challenges and strengths. In N. G. Johnson, M. C. Roberts, & J. Worell (Ed.), *Beyond appearance: A new look at adolescent girls* (pp. 151-174). Washington, DC: American Psychological Association.

Walcott, D. D., Pratt, H. D., & Patel, D. R. (2003). Adolescents and eating disorders: Gender, racial, ethnic, sociocultural, and socioeconomic issues. *Journal of Adolescent Research, 18*(3), 223-243.

Wildes, J. E., Emery, R. E., & Simons, A. D. (2001). The roles of ethnicity and culture in the development of eating disturbance and body dissatisfaction: A meta-analytic review. *Clinical Psychology Review, 21*(4), 521-551.

Wooley, S. C. (1994). Sexual abuse and eating disorders: The concealed debate. In P. Fallon, M. A. Katzman, & S. C. Wooley (Eds.), *Feminist perspectives on eating disorders* (pp. 171-211). New York: Guilford.

doi:10.1300/J015v30n03_13

Group Counseling with Asian American Women: Reflections and Effective Practices

Yuli Liu
Yuying Tsong
Diane Hayashino

SUMMARY. This article presents culturally specific practices with counseling Asian American women in the group modality. Using a theoretical framework that integrates multiculturalism and feminism, this article offers collective reflections from three Asian American female therapists and their experiences as facilitators of two Asian American women's groups on a college campus. The overall structure, design, and format of the groups are discussed, from recruitment, screening, and conducting the first session to termination. Central themes such as identity and value conflicts, as well as dynamics within the two Asian American women's groups are also illustrated. Lastly, limitations to the observations presented in this article are discussed. doi:10.1300/J015v30n03_14

Yuli Liu, PhD, is Staff Psychologist, Counseling Center at University of California, Riverside. Yuying Tsong, PhD, is Program Chair in the Counseling Psychology Ed.D. Program at Argosy University. Diane Hayashino, PhD, is Staff Psychologist at the Counseling and Psychological Services at California State University, Long Beach.

Address correspondence to: Yuli Liu, Veitch Student Center, North Wing, University of California, Riverside, Riverside, CA 92521 (E-mail: yuli.liu@ucr.edu).

[Haworth co-indexing entry note]: "Group Counseling with Asian American Women: Reflections and Effective Practices." Liu, Yuli, Yuying Tsong, and Diane Hayashino. Co-published simultaneously in *Women & Therapy* (The Haworth Press, Inc.) Vol. 30, No. 3/4, 2007, pp. 193-208; and: *Feminist Reflections on Growth and Transformation: Asian American Women in Therapy* (ed: Debra M. Kawahara, and Oliva M. Espín) The Haworth Press, Inc., 2007, pp. 193-208. Single or multiple copies of this article are available for a fee from The Haworth Document Delivery Service [1-800-HAWORTH, 9:00 a.m. - 5:00 p.m. (EST). E-mail address: docdelivery@haworthpress.com].

Available online at http://wt.haworthpress.com

doi:10.1300/J015v30n03_14

KEYWORDS. Asian American, Asian American women, group therapy, culturally specific counseling, multicultural counseling, gender issues

> Asian and Asian American women on the whole struggle with multiple forces in order to achieve belonging in a multicultural environment. These struggles can have significant emotional sequelae that are appropriate for psychotherapeutic attention. (Bradshaw, 1994)

The number of Asian American women pursuing a college education in the U.S. is growing rapidly. According to the U.S. Census in 2000, Asian Americans comprise approximately 4.2 percent of the U.S. population. Asian Americans make up approximately six percent of all students in higher education, with women making up approximately 51 percent of all Asian American students (Wilds, 2000). These women represent an extremely diverse group in terms of immigration history, generation level, language, religion, socioeconomic status, values, and ethnic specific experiences. College is a significant time for many students, as this is typically the first experience of being separated from home. They may struggle with being physically away from home while the values of family obligation and loyalty remain intact. Particularly for Asian American women, the developmental issues of balancing academics, family, and interpersonal relationships can sometimes leave them feeling overwhelmed and confused, and often lead to more serious mental health issues such as depression and anxiety (Wong & Mock, 1997). The diversity of Asian American women college students must be acknowledged and addressed in the provision of culturally appropriate mental health services on college campuses.

Past literature on culturally specific services primarily focused on individual rather than group therapy interventions. The research is sparse on the effectiveness of group therapy as a treatment modality for Asian Americans. Yu and Gregg (1993) noted that group counseling with Asian American clients is not the same as facilitating traditional Western groups. For some Asian American clients, traditional group therapy approaches that emphasize verbalization, confrontation, individuation, conflict resolution, and autonomy may be confusing and lead to premature termination. Tsui (1997) reported that homogeneous Asian therapy groups are beneficial in ensuring a degree of comfort and familiarity that facilitates discussion and sharing. On the other hand, given within- and between-group differences evident in Asian and Asian American groups, issues of boundaries, sociopolitical identity, and confidentiality may impede the process of group therapy. Group facilitators must not only be sensitive and aware of the differences among members' ethnic backgrounds, they must have the multicultural knowledge, skills, and awareness to handle these issues.

Asian Americans historically tend to underutilize traditional mental health services. Rather than interpret these findings as support for the "model minority" myth, it is important that we explore the complexity and diversity of the Asian American experience, issues such as oppression and racism, sexism, acculturation, and identity development. Uba (1994) identified various barriers to accessing mental health services for Asian Americans. One of the significant barriers is the cultural inhibition about seeking services, specifically the stigma attached to mental health problems, the shame on the family, and the inadequate identification of mental health issues. Additional barriers include the lack of financial resources, geographical inaccessibility, the lack of knowledge of available services, and a shortage of culturally sensitive and bilingual staff. Given that Asian Americans tend to delay initial contact for counseling services, have higher attrition rates, and a shorter duration of therapy, the need for culturally specific services cannot be ignored. More current studies reveal that Asian Americans' preference for counseling styles may differ from the assumptions of Western psychotherapies (Byon, Chan, & Thomas, 1999). Additionally, research indicated that Asian Americans utilize mental health services as often as other groups, particularly when services are culturally sensitive to their needs as well as strengths (Akutsu, 1997). Fujino, Okazaki, and Young's (1994) study suggested that ethnic and gender match between Asian American women and their therapists reduces premature termination and increases duration of treatment. Thus, providing an Asian American Women's group with Asian American women facilitators on a college campus serves to challenge some of the barriers. It also utilizes participants' and facilitators' strengths, increases access to counseling and contributes to culturally competent mental health services.

The purpose of this article is to share the collective experiences as facilitators of two Asian American Women's groups on a college campus. The three facilitators are Asian American women who have been trained in programs that emphasize grounding in multicultural counseling competencies. In order to achieve such grounding, our training has included taking interdisciplinary courses, participating in adult and child practica within culturally diverse communities, conducting community-based research, and engaging in critical thinking through dialogues with colleagues as well as with each other. We are from different ethnic and generational backgrounds, including a third generation Japanese American, a "1.5" generation Taiwanese American, and a first generation Taiwanese American. We value the integration of our personal and professional identities to allow for flexibility in our role as psychologists. Facilitating these groups requires a balance of self-exploration and creative vision in developing culturally specific group interventions.

THEORETICAL FOUNDATION

The facilitators share a similar theoretical foundation of integrated feminism and multiculturalism. Although sexism is a factor in the lives of women of color, it is crucial to be aware of the difficulties and oppression that accompany racism. Many women of color have worked simultaneously for civil rights and women's rights and understand the need for a connection between civil rights and feminism. For many women of color, racism is a far more visible, powerful, and day-to-day experience than sexism. At the same time, the oppression within some Asian American patriarchical cultures remains personal and potent, since these communities are based on a structured hierarchy of gender, age, generation, with well-defined gender roles and family roles (Chow, 1991). Thus, it is essential in working with Asian American women to integrate both feminism and multiculturalism as well as to recognize the complexity of the intersection of culture and gender in their lives.

We have an inclusive definition of feminism that is very similar to one noted by bell hooks (1981) who views feminism as a commitment to eliminating all forms of oppression, including racism, sexism, heterosexism, and classism. Enns (1997) also shares a similar view that a competent feminist counselor understands that effective feminist therapy is based on an ongoing and continuous examination of personal values, intentional creation of an approach that demonstrates consistency between one's theoretical orientation to feminism and theoretical approach to psychotherapy, and an understanding of how intersections of gender, race, class, economic status, and sexual orientation influence women's and men's lives. We agree with Reynolds' (2001) definition of multiculturalism from both universal and race-based perspectives. She believes that the full range of social identities that influence who we are (race, class, gender, sexual orientation, religion, abilities, and age) have to be understood and incorporated into our understanding of multiculturalism. All the experiences from the perspectives of these social identities shape who we are and how we relate to others.

Corey (2001) supports the integration of feminism and multiculturalism and acknowledges that feminist and multicultural approaches to counseling share many common principles. Both approaches place an emphasis on considering who the counselor is as a person and her impact on the counseling relationship, acknowledging and valuing multiple aspects of the client's identity, and creating a therapeutic alliance that allows the client to work collaboratively with the counselor in choosing an appropriate intervention (Nishimura, 2004). Espin (1994) wrote that ethnic specific therapy provides several advantages, including: the therapist can understand the ethnicity of the client from "first-hand experience" and the therapist is more likely to be invested in the client's progress in therapy.

In working with the Asian American women in our groups, we do not present as the authority in solving issues related to being Asian American women. Rather, we honor the multiple identities and experiences of each client by engaging in a collaborative relationship with mutually defined goals that are appropriate to each client's personality and psychological developmental level. We also strive to create an egalitarian relationship and a working alliance that can empower our clients and acknowledge the multiple roles and identities they have in their lives. Lastly, we consistently process and acknowledge our own beliefs and attitudes about racism, sexism, classism, heterosexism, religions, and family dynamics (e.g., filial piety, divorce, extramarital relationships, interracial dating and marriage, and premarital sex).

OVERALL STRUCTURE OF THE ASIAN AMERICAN WOMEN'S GROUP

An initial step in developing culturally specific groups is designing the group to address the significant barriers to seeking counseling services in all aspects of the group structure, from recruitment, screening, opening and closing of the sessions, and co-facilitators' debriefing. In preparing to form an Asian American Women's group, several issues arise that pertain to the recruitment of members, the screening process, the structure of the group, and introductory and termination sessions. In addition, it is extremely important to debrief as co-facilitators throughout the group process to discuss our reactions and countertransference toward the group that may stem from our own biases and experiences. Due to the diverse ethnic groups under the "Asian American" umbrella term, we find that it is crucial to recognize any limitations in our knowledge and skills working with clients of certain ethnicities or religions. We seek to fill this void through consultation and learning more about these populations through the group members and additional research. While intentionally structuring the Asian American Women's group to be culturally responsive, we hope to increase the utilization of counseling services and prevent premature termination.

Recruitment

The advertising and naming of the group are important matters to consider as the group may draw certain students and exclude others. As ethnic identity is one of the main issues for Asian American women, the very act of seeking to join a group of racially similar women is intricately tied to one's identity. For students who have a more traditionally defined ethnic identity, they may not feel comfortable attending an "Asian American" women's group versus an Asian women's group or an ethnic specific organization. Conversely, highly acculturated or marginalized Asian American women may also choose not to be associated with a group that clearly focuses on racial and cultural group memberships. Biracial or multiracial women may also express concerns regarding a sense of belonging to the group as they come from multiple heritages. Group facilitators must take the implied inclusivity of the group into consideration when naming the group. Both of the groups that we facilitated were named the "Asian American Women's Group," while other group names such as "Asian Pacific Islander Women's Support Group" or "Asian American Women's Forum" can also be considered.

Recognizing that stigma may be associated with seeking counseling services (Uba, 1994), flyers were also designed to highlight the discussion of common issues facing college students and Asian American women, rather than a focus on mental health problems. While our groups met at the university counseling center, other locations that are more neutral can be considered, such as a women's resource center or a cross-cultural center. Through advertising flyers, emails, and active outreach and promotion of the group by making contact with student organizations, academic units, and other student affairs departments, co-facilitators can normalize help-seeking and encourage women who identify as Asian, Asian American, Pacific Islander, biracial, or multiracial to attend the group. Referrals from counseling center staff members and from direct outreach and advertising were the main sources of referrals for our groups.

Screenings

Like other process groups, an individual screening meeting is an important step to ensure that the potential group member is a good fit for the group. It is also an opportunity for co-facilitators to address concerns students may have about the group, and to provide an introduction to the process of counseling and group counseling. Based on the screening, counseling strategies can be modified to the needs of the group members and their receptivity to counseling. In discussing the purpose of the Asian American women's group, co-facilitators may also assess the student's presenting concerns for relevant cultural factors and match between the student's issues and the goals of the group.

Co-facilitators may utilize an intake format that pays particular attention to the potential member's ethnic heritage, immigration history, acculturation level, generational status, ethnic identity, sexual orientation, religion, gender role, and socioeconomic status. Potential members are also encouraged to think about goals they have for the group experience and what they expect to occur in the group process. Similar to other process groups, co-facilitators must be attuned to factors that may exclude someone from joining the group or fully benefiting from the group, such as a high risk of danger to self or others, psychotic symptoms, or personality disorders. Co-facilitators are prepared to make appropriate referrals to individual counseling and/or medication evaluation when necessary. Lastly, when co-facilitators have agreed that the potential group member is appropriate for the group, group norms such as regular attendance and confidentiality are reviewed in preparation for the group experience.

In our experience with individual screenings, we also found it helpful in connecting with students to share our own ethnic backgrounds and reasons we are committed to offering this group. By doing so, we communicate our value for each member's unique experience as an Asian American woman. We also found that students often mentioned their comfort level with other Asian American women, which we incorporated into discussions about identity and expectations for joining the group. Therefore, it was crucial that we emphasized in our screenings the value for the female perspective. We found screening meetings to be quite important in preparing students for the group counseling experience, preparing ourselves for potential themes to discuss in group, and shaping the composition of the group.

Format of the Group

Given the time-limited nature of counseling services across college campuses, therapy groups also tend to be short-term and follow a quarter or semester timeframe. We have observed Asian American Women's groups on other college campuses structured in several different ways, for example, as open-ended drop-in support groups, as closed process groups with screenings, and as time-limited structured groups with weekly predetermined topics. The number of group members may also vary, as we have had groups comprised of between 5 to 10 women. The structure of the group needs to be flexible and reflect not only the goals of the co-facilitators, but the needs of the group members as well. For example, co-facilitators of a closed process group will need to survey members of the group regarding their input when new members wish to join the group. The two groups that we conducted were short-term (8-12 sessions), met weekly for 90 minute sessions, and were closed process groups with screened members.

First Session

The first session of the Asian American women's group is crucial for welcoming and introducing members, as well as reviewing and developing group norms and cohesion. In addition to self-introductions about members' status in school and their majors, women in the group are also encouraged to share their ethnic background, generational status, family immigration history, birth order, religion, and other information they believe is pertinent. Co-facilitators also model for members by sharing their own backgrounds and what their roles will be in the group. This invites members to consider the impact of culture and gender in their lives. Typically, themes begin to emerge during group members' introductions and the co-facilitators can start to process and explore these connections within the group. Co-facilitators also focus on here-and-now dynamics and encourage members to process their feelings regarding attending the first group meeting, such as anxiety, awkwardness, or excitement. In doing so, we can appropriately model for group members the need to address reactions in the group. While group norms such as respect, prompt and regular attendance, and confidentiality are discussed during the first session, group members are also invited to create other norms that will contribute to a meaningful group experience. At the conclusion of the first session, co-facilitators ask the women to share thoughts and reflections on their experience of the first group meeting.

The first session typically required more structure from the co-facilitators to set up the group norms and to facilitate the members' self-introductions and initial interactions. For example, in one group, the facilitators gave each member a piece of paper with a stick figure drawn on it and asked the members to write down the "labels" or "images" that come to mind when they think of the term "Asian American women." We included prompts such as age, height, weight, ethnicity, area born and raised, language spoken at home, religious and/or spiritual influences, sexual orientation, socioeconomic status, and career interests. This exercise helped the members to start talking about their common and different views and perceptions about Asian American women and how they see themselves as an Asian American woman.

Termination

Participation in the Asian American women's group is often an emotional and meaningful journey for the women involved. We have found that the impending termination may signify loss, change, satisfaction, or loneliness, among other feelings, for the women in the group. Termination is discussed in advance with the group. Some groups may wish to have a celebratory ritual, such as a potluck, to signify the end of the group and the work they have accomplished. Group members, including the co-facilitators, may also publicly acknowledge how they have impacted each other and what it means to say good-bye. Some group members exchange contact information and plan to keep in touch after termination. While the co-facilitators and group members may determine the actual format of the termination session, its significance for providing closure to a powerful experience in connecting with racially similar women cannot be overlooked.

The termination sessions in both of our groups were significant and memorable experiences. We found that it was important to plan in advance with the facilitators as well as group members about how they wanted to mark this occasion. In one group, the facilitators addressed each member of the group and reflected upon her growth in the group, then invited everyone to share thoughts and feelings about themselves, others, and the group process. Facilitators emphasized each member's strengths, empowering her to become the "expert" in her experience.

CONTENT AND PROCESS OF GROUP

While the structure and format of our groups are important considerations to effective group practices, the themes and dynamics or the content and process of the group also deserve attention. We will share our collective observations and reflections on the central themes that emerged in both groups, as well as our observations regarding the group process. The content and process of the groups represent an applied understanding of the integration of the multicultural and feminist theoretical approaches.

Central Themes in Group

The validation of shared experiences and feelings among group members contributes to a sense of universality within the group. One of the main themes of the group was a discussion of their identities, and the impact of their identities on interpersonal relationships, including family relationships. While group members ranged from those who have recently immigrated to those who are second generation and beyond, many discussed the tug between values from their cultures of origin and Western/American values. The group was a place for the women to examine sources that have had the strongest influences on the formation of their values and identity, including parents, ethnic community, peers, educational institution, and the media. Depending on the acculturation levels of group members, some also expressed shame in being unable to speak the same language as their parents, or embarrassment about coming to counseling. There may also be ambivalence about revealing family "secrets," such as abuse, extramarital affairs, or domestic violence, given many Asian cultures' emphasis on maintaining honor or "face" for one's family. Other issues in the Asian American women's group included experiences with racism, sexism, and discrimination, in settings such as work and school. Group members also examined their own internalized racism, such as discomfort with their skin color or ethnic features, or dislike of more recent Asian immigrants. The Asian American women's group provided a safe environment for women to explore the different aspects of their identities and to learn from the diversity of identities in other group members.

The group also served as a resource for women to discuss how to balance internal struggles and external conflicts with family members. These value conflicts are often inherent in intergenerational conflicts with parents, disclosures regarding family functioning, dilemmas over choosing a major or career, conflicts over choice of dating or marriage partners, and seeking a balance between school/work and family. Another theme that emerged is linked to these women's identities, in that conflicts emerged when these women made "unconventional" choices regarding their decisions, whether it was to pursue a career deemed atypical for Asian Americans, or to date/marry someone from a different ethnic background. At times, group members making these "unconventional" decisions faced the prospects of losing their family's or community's support and validation. It was often common for the women in the groups to be supportive of each other's struggles and reaffirm their strengths in overcoming adversity.

Process Observations

In addition to the central themes from the group sessions, we also observed themes at the group process level. While group members formed bonds with each other quickly, they also had conflicts with each other because of their differences and/or similarities in acculturation, generational status, roles in the family, socioeconomic status, and religion. As discussed above, issues concerning the family were one of the central themes in the group discussions, and we found that some of the group members would often have conflicted views and disagree when the discussions involved family roles (e.g., filial piety, children's responsibilities to parents, younger siblings' deference to the older siblings). We find this "reenactment" of family roles to be more salient in our Asian American Women's group than the other women's group we have led. We speculate that one of the reasons may have to do with the more structured and hierarchical family roles, and the importance of "roles" in the identity formation of Asian American women.

Different from the traditional psychotherapy group of mixed race/ethnicities, we also found that group members tended to seek advice from group facilitators more frequently, possibly as a function of viewing co-facilitators as authorities. Initially, the group members tended to wait for facilitators to lead and/or direct the group. As the group continued, their ability to process with one another deepened since many of the group members made contact with each other outside of the group session. In fact, many of the group members continued to maintain contact with each other following termination.

An observation of the group process that is consistent with the literature (Uba, 1994) is the role of stigma toward seeking mental health. Some of the members expressed their concerns in seeking individual therapy during or after group counseling, because they felt that being in a group is similar to being in a discussion group and not the same as participating in "psychological treatment." Seeking individual therapy means admitting "there is something wrong with me." We also heard the opposite views toward group counseling. Some of the group members shared that it was more difficult for them to disclose in a group setting, especially at the beginning, because they thought individual therapy would be more private. The ability to explore group members' shame regarding seeking counseling was a common issue addressed in the group. However, at the end of the group, most of the group members indicated that they were more open and felt less shame towards seeking individual and group therapy.

REFLECTIONS AND EFFECTIVE PRACTICES IN LEADING ASIAN AMERICAN WOMEN'S GROUPS

Adopting the philosophy of multiculturalism and feminism in leading the Asian American Women's group, we identify certain practices to be effective in contributing to the growth of the group. Our experience as facilitators for the Asian American Women's group is unique from facilitating other non-culturally specific therapy groups. Culturally specific services include aspects such as recognizing the family as an integral part of therapy, establishing a personal therapeutic relationship, addressing issues of shame, reevaluating the meaning of self, and recognizing the benefits of a cultural therapeutic milieu (Zane, Hatanaka, Park, & Akutsu, 1994). We want to identify and describe how some of these aspects are apparent and how they might contribute to the group experience.

Different from traditional psychotherapy process groups, the group facilitators are more flexible regarding boundaries with the group members. This is consistent with our feminist and multicultural orientations as therapists (Enns, 2000). We actively seek to foster openness and trust in the group with our own self-disclosures about appropriate experiences related to our gender and ethnicity. For example, to validate the experience of balancing multiple roles in her family, one of the facilitators shared how, at times, she felt isolated from her family as she pursued her graduate degree. We also experienced the importance of flexibility in terms of our multiple roles as a counselor, considering the potential risks for exploitation and harm, according to ethical guidelines. For example, we found ourselves serving as mentors to some of the members after the group terminated. Some of the group members went on to work with us in different non-clinical capacities at the university and consulted us about applying to graduate schools. There was also less restriction of "gift giving" than in traditional therapy groups. For example, when one of the group facilitators graduated from her doctoral program, the group members decided to give her a small graduation gift to celebrate the milestone. This led into a discussion of the multiple factors impacting their career choices. These boundary issues require ongoing consultation regarding our ethical responsibilities as a counselor. Boundaries among group members themselves were also more fluid and open. Often the women opted to exchange contact information outside of the group to continue supporting each other, or to offer resources to each other (such as suggested readings or announcements about community events). While we emphasized confidentiality about discussing what was shared in the group, we did not discourage these outside contacts as they tended to strengthen the cohesiveness of the group.

Another practice that is effective in facilitating an Asian American women's group is to encourage the women to understand their issues within the broader context of culture, gender, and society. In providing a broader systemic perspective, women in the group are more aware of the impact of racism, patriarchy, and the messages that they have internalized as a result of these societal influences. Co-facilitators also encouraged women in the group to examine from where and from whom they have learned their values. By contextualizing their experiences, co-facilitators sought to empower these women to begin working against negative internalized messages about what it means to be a woman of color.

During the process of forming the Asian American Women's group, the co-facilitators also paid attention to the composition of the group, and how group members from different age groups, ethnicities, acculturation levels, socioeconomic statuses, and generational statuses might fit together. We wanted to create a supportive environment that recognizes the heterogeneity of the Asian American women's experience. As co-facilitators, we also are aware of our presumed roles as "experts" and balance group members' needs for advice with using the other women in the group as a resource.

LIMITATIONS

There are several limitations to the findings and observations we present in this article. First, the Asian American women in the groups were college students from a university with 60% of Asian American Pacific Islander (AAPI) students. Therefore, their experiences may be different from those Asian American women who attend schools with a smaller percentage of AAPI students. Second, the Asian American Women's Groups took place at a college counseling center setting with mostly traditional college age students (18 to 25 years old). Third, the group facilitators share the same heterosexual orientation, and did not explicitly explore members' sexual orientations, which may or may not contribute to the lack of discussion on this aspect of their identity. Recognizing the inherent reservations around issues of sexuality and sexual orientation due to traditional gender roles in Asian cultures (Aoki, 1997), co-facilitators note the need to be more proactive in addressing these issues to be fully inclusive of the intersections of culture, gender, and sexual orientation for the women in our groups. Fourth, while a wide range of issues was discussed in our groups, there was a lack of discussion of sexuality. Almost all of the group members shared the difficulties they experience in having or not having boyfriends, yet they rarely discussed issues related to sexuality. Fifth, the Asian American Women's groups we presented in this article were conducted based on the short-term therapy model (8 to 12 sessions), which in itself has its limitations. Almost all group members at termination indicated that they would have liked more group sessions as they started to explore more of themselves. Lastly, we identified the group as an Asian American Women's group, which may have unintentionally alienated or discouraged participation from Pacific Islander or other AAPI students who do not identify as "Asian American" on campus.

CONCLUSION

These culturally specific strategies serve to highlight the need to work with Asian American women within a cultural context that is sensitive to the intersection of gender and ethnicity. It is crucial that applied research continues to address the therapy needs and conditions that Asian American women face. Based on our experiences, we found these strategies to be effective in the growth of the Asian American women's group. As Asian American women, our experiences as facilitators were extremely rewarding and we were honored to be able to offer culturally specific services to the Asian American community on campus. With this article, we wish not only to challenge the barriers Asian American women face in seeking mental health services, but also to highlight their strengths by utilizing a multicultural and feminist framework as a viable therapeutic modality in working with Asian American women.

REFERENCES

Akutsu, P. (1997). Mental health care delivery to Asian Americans: Review of the literature. In E. Lee (Ed.), *Working with Asian Americans: A guide for clinicians* (pp. 464-475). New York: Guilford Press.

Aoki, B. (1997). Gay and lesbian Asian Americans in psychotherapy. In E. Lee (Ed.), *Working with Asian Americans: A guide for clinicians* (pp. 411-419). New York: Guilford Press.

Bradshaw, C. (1994). Asian and Asian American women: Historical and political considerations in psychotherapy. In L. Comas-Diaz & B. Greene (Eds.), *Women of color: Integrating ethnic and gender identities in psychotherapy* (pp. 72-113). New York: Guilford Press.

Byon, K., Chan, F., & Thomas, K. (1999). Korean international students' expectations about counseling. *Journal of College Counseling, 2*, 99-109.

Chow, E. (1991). The development of feminist consciousness among Asian American women. In J. Lorber & S. A. Fatrell (Eds.), *The social construction of gender* (pp. 255-268). Newbury Park, CA: Sage.

Corey, G. (2001). *The art of integrative counseling*. Belmont, CA: Brooks/Cole.

Enns, C. (1997). *Feminist theories and feminist psychotherapies: Origins, themes, and variations*. New York: The Haworth Press, Inc.

Enns, C. (2000). Gender issues in counseling. In S. D. Brown & R. W. Lent (Eds.), *Handbook of counseling psychology* (pp. 601-638). New York: Wiley & Sons.

Espin, O. (1994). Feminist approaches. In L. Comas-Diaz & B. Greene (Eds.), *Women of color: Integrating ethnic and gender identities in psychotherapy* (pp. 265-286). New York: Guilford Press.

Fujino, D., Okazaki, S., & Young, K. (1994). Asian-American women in the mental health system: An examination of ethnic and gender match between therapist and client. *Journal of Community Psychology, 22*(2), 164-176.

hooks, b. (1981). *Ain't I a woman*. Boston: South End Press.

Nishimura, N. (2004). Counseling biracial women: An intersection of multiculturalism and feminism. *Women & Therapy, 27*(1/2), 133-145.

Reynolds, A. (2001). Embracing multiculturalism: A journey of self-discovery. In J. G. Ponterotto, J. M. Casas, L. A. Suzuki, & C. M. Alexander (Eds.), *Handbook of multicultural counseling* (2nd ed., pp. 103-112). Thousand Oaks, CA: Sage.

Tsui, P. (1997). The dynamics of cultural and power relations in group therapy. In E. Lee (Ed.), *Working with Asian Americans: A guide for clinicians* (pp. 354-363). New York: Guilford Press.

Uba, L. (1994). *Asian Americans: Personality patterns, identity and mental health.* New York: Guilford Press.

Wilds, D. (2000). *Minorities in higher education 1999-2000: Seventeenth annual status report.* Washington, DC: American Council on Education.

Wong, L., & Mock, M. (1997). Asian American young adults. In E. Lee (Ed.), *Working with Asian Americans: A guide for clinicians* (pp. 196-207). New York: Guilford Press.

Yu, A., & Gregg, C. (1993). Asians in groups: More than a matter of cultural awareness. *The Journal for Specialists in Group Work, 18*(2), 86-93.

Zane, N., Hatanaka, H., Park, S., & Akutsu, P. (1994). Ethnic-specific mental health services: Evaluation of the parallel approach for Asian-American clients. *Journal of Community Psychology, 22*, 68-81.

doi:10.1300/J015v30n03_14

TRAINING

Training Therapists to Be Culturally Sensitive with Asian American Women Clients

Karen L. Suyemoto
Joan H. Liem
with
Jennifer C. Kuhn
Elizabeth A. Mongillo
Jesse J. Tauriac

SUMMARY. We describe here a developmental sequence of three key training experiences that contribute to developing cultural sensitivity for

Karen L. Suyemoto, PhD, is Assistant Professor, Psychology Department and Joan H. Liem, PhD, is Associate Professor of Psychology, University of Massachusetts, Boston.

Address correspondence to: Karen L. Suyemoto, PhD, Assistant Professor or Joan H. Liem, PhD, Associate Professor, Psychology Dept., University of Massachusetts, Boston, MA 02125-3393 USA (E-mail: karen.suyemoto@umb.edu) or (joan.liem@umb.edu).

[Haworth co-indexing entry note]: "Training Therapists to Be Culturally Sensitive with Asian American Women Clients." Suyemoto, Karen L., and Joan H. Liem. Co-published simultaneously in *Women & Therapy* (The Haworth Press, Inc.) Vol. 30, No. 3/4, 2007, pp. 209-227; and: *Feminist Reflections on Growth and Transformation: Asian American Women in Therapy* (ed: Debra M. Kawahara, and Oliva M. Espín) The Haworth Press, Inc., 2007, pp. 209-227. Single or multiple copies of this article are available for a fee from The Haworth Document Delivery Service [1-800-HAWORTH, 9:00 a.m. - 5:00 p.m. (EST). E-mail address: docdelivery@haworthpress.com].

Available online at http://wt.haworthpress.com

doi:10.1300/J015v30n03_15

clinicians who are not of Asian heritage and are working with Asian American women. The sequence reflects and illustrates our guiding assumptions for developing multicultural sensitivity, including an emphasis on cultural self-awareness and a reflexive approach to knowledge acquisition and clinical practice. Effects of these training experiences are illustrated through three case examples of therapy with Asian American women written by an African American male and two European American female therapists at different stages in their training. doi:10.1300/J015v30n03_15 *[Article copies available for a fee from The Haworth Document Delivery Service: 1-800-HAWORTH. E-mail address: <docdelivery@haworthpress.com> Website: <http://www.HaworthPress.com>*

KEYWORDS. Graduate psychology education, multicultural education, psychotherapy education, Asian American, women, therapy

Most therapy with Asian American women is provided by therapists who are not Asian American women. Although a burgeoning literature describes their mental health needs, Asian American women continue to confront barriers to receiving culturally sensitive care. These include clinicians' lack of knowledge about the worldviews of diverse cultural groups, tendencies to view differences as pathological, and lack of culturally sensitive skills, resulting in biased or inappropriate treatment. To address these barriers, multicultural psychologists emphasize the need for service providers to: increase their awareness and understanding of their own racial and cultural experiences; become knowledgeable about the experiences of clients from backgrounds different from their own; and develop skills that are culturally sensitive. However, it is not always clear *how* to develop increased cultural self-awareness and understanding of others, or culturally competent clinical skills. This article describes training experiences aimed at developing culturally sensitive professional practice, particularly as it is related to clinical work with Asian American women when the therapist is not Asian American.

FOUNDATIONS OF TRAINING TO WORK WITH ASIAN AMERICAN WOMEN

Guiding Assumptions for Developing Multicultural Sensitivity

In addition to adopting a sociocultural perspective on health and psychopathology, acquiring multicultural sensitivity requires an ongoing commitment to self-exploration and a reflexive approach to knowledge acquisition and clinical practice. Students in scientist/practitioner psychology programs enter their training with wide-ranging prior exposure to different cultures, and varying degrees of awareness related to their own and others' experiences linked to gender, race, culture, class background, and the privilege or oppression associated with these statuses. Our training model assumes that cultural sensitivity and clinical competence are developed over time in the context of increasingly challenging learning experiences (see American Psychological Association, 2003 and Arredondo et al., 1996, for operationalization and evaluation of cultural sensitivity). Trainees are first exposed to new information about themselves as cultural beings within systems of power and privilege and are encouraged to explore the meaning of the new information in light of prior experiences and values. Trainees are then exposed to and expected to seek out information intended to further their understanding of the cultural identities and social positions of diverse others. Over time, this new information becomes integrated into their worldviews and personal and professional identities, and translates into actions, including more culturally sensitive clinical interventions. This integration further enhances cultural self-awareness and reflexivity and fuels the motivation to learn more. It is not enough for a training program to initiate this learning process, it must also continually cultivate it in all aspects of training, including academic coursework, research training, and supervised clinical practice.

We stress self-awareness because we believe that one's own experiences with gender, race, and culture; one's own positions of relative power and privilege; and one's own unconscious or unintentional biases rooted in racism, ethnocentrism, or sexism inherently affect one's professional activities. Without this self-awareness, clinicians may unintentionally enact racial or gender biases within their roles as therapists, and may thus perpetuate the biases within the field that contribute to barriers to care. Reflexivity contributes to the understanding that oppression and bias are systemic problems that are socialized within people whether or not they desire to benefit from or participate in these systems. It encourages a critical perspective and fosters the motivation to work continually on the development of cultural sensitivity in the ongoing teaching/learning/application cycle described above.

Foundational Understandings of Asian American Women

One challenge in developing culturally sensitive training about Asian American women is determining how much to emphasize similarities across ethnic groups (particularly in contrast to the dominant discourse about women that unreflectively references White European American women), and how much to emphasize the heterogeneity of each ethnic group of Asian American women. Because the majority of Asian American women are from immigrant families (immigrants themselves or children of immigrants), their cultures of origin frequently have more influence on their current functioning than is typically the case for most European Americans who have greater generational distance from their original ethnic culture(s). Many Asian American women experience issues related to intergenerational conflicts, marital stresses due to changing gender roles, tensions associated with negotiating family and career responsibilities and desires, and related domestic violence (see, e.g., Chin, 2000; Chung, 2001; Eng, 1995; Root, 1995, 1998; Sue & Sue, 2002). Many Asian American refugee women also experience symptoms associated with war and flight, including experiencing or witnessing assault, rape, starvation, childbirth in traumatic circumstances, and/or the violent deaths of close family members (Thai, 2002; Uba, 1994). Many Asian American women also experience a lack of familiarity with mental health concepts and practices within their cultures, different ways of conceptualizing and treating mental health issues than those employed in the U.S., and a reluctance to use mental health services due to the lack of cultural sensitivity in service providers and the stigma associated with psychological illness prevalent in their communities (Sue & Sue; Uba; U.S. Department of Health and Human Services, 2001). Most Asian American women also share experiences related to racial and ethnic discrimination in the United States–whether this is consciously or unconsciously enacted or experienced–including: stereotyping of women of Asian descent as exotic, assumptions about Asian American women's personality traits (e.g., their submissiveness) or abilities (e.g. their lack of English language proficiency), or racial profiling related to their assumed gang affiliation (Root; Uba).

However, while Asian American women share some experiences, they are an extremely heterogeneous group, including women from different generations within the United States and representing 29-32 different ethnic/subgroup backgrounds varying in language, values, and other aspects of culture (Atkinson, Morten, & Sue, 1998). These women vary widely in their adherence to traditional "Asian" values and behaviors, their knowledge about and comfort with U.S. values and behaviors, and their awareness of the impact of race and ethnicity on their social experiences and the ways in which others perceive them (Root, 1995, 1998; Uba, 1994). Each

Asian American woman also has specific personal and familial experiences and negotiates specific contexts that make her unique.

Thus, those training to work with Asian American women clients must simultaneously develop: (1) understanding of the modal experiences of Asian Americans as a racial and pan-ethnic group in comparison with the dominant European American group and the socially constructed nature of this experience; (2) some comparative exposure to the modal experiences of women (as opposed to men) from different Asian American ethnic groups as well as comparative understandings about how each group differs from another; and (3) simultaneous consideration and awareness of the multiple variables that create differences *within* each group. Because it is impossible to teach trainees all they need to know to treat all Asian American women clients, it is imperative to teach them a process of learning that can be used to gather information and guide them in creating culturally sensitive interventions in their future work.

We describe here a developmental sequence of three key training experiences in the first through third years of a clinical psychology program, focusing on the influence of this training on non-Asian student therapists' emerging cultural sensitivity and therapeutic skill development as they pertain to working with Asian American women.

INTRODUCING CULTURAL SENSITIVITY AND SELF-AWARENESS: CULTURE AND MENTAL HEALTH

Culture and Mental Health (CMH) is required of students in their first semester of their first year. In our developmental understanding of training for cultural sensitivity, the course aims to provide basic information that introduces trainees to the complexities of race and culture (and intersections with gender, class, sexual orientation, and disability: see Weber, 1998). It addresses these issues not only as individual experiences, but also as systems of privilege and oppression that inherently affect one's worldview and are reflected in the history and current structure of psychology and psychotherapy. It introduces students to research and theory relevant to working with racial minorities and encourages a critical analysis of this literature. It aims to develop students' awareness of their own experiences and positions in these systems and integrates these understandings into their current worldviews, thus enhancing their commitment to developing cultural sensitivity as part of their professional identities.

Understanding and Treating Asian American Women

The major challenges for trainees who are not Asian American in understanding and treating Asian American women at this point in their training are: (1) their lack of information about Asian American women (and their diversity) that contributes to stereotyping or overgeneralization and; (2) their general lack of self-awareness in relation to how their own experiences of race, culture, gender, and other systems of power and privilege shape their worldviews, perceptions of others, clinical conceptualizations, and therapeutic choices.

In some ways, students' lack of knowledge about Asian American women seems easy to address. Information about Asian American women is presented in readings, films (see the National Asian American Telecommunications Association for films about Asian Americans: www.naatanet.org), and discussions in CMH and other classes throughout the training program. However, difficulties in meeting this challenge lie in avoiding overgeneralization, oversimplification, and reification of oppressive categorizations through: (1) balancing modal information with consideration of heterogeneity, (2) placing research, theory, and application within the sociopolitical and socio-historical contexts of systemic privilege, and (3) encouraging critical analysis of the socially constructed meanings of these variables and the ways in which psychological research, theory, and practice have engaged them. For example, in CMH, although readings addressing modal experiences of Asian Americans are assigned and discussed, personal narratives of Asian American women are also included to emphasize the heterogeneity of the group (e.g., see Cox, 1999; Lee, 1992). The existing literature is also critiqued, particularly in relation to generalizations and stereotypes about Asian Americans and consideration given to Asian American women who don't fit within the more researched East Asian "model minority" such as multiracial, adopted, South Asian, or Southeast Asian refugee women. While issues well-researched in psychology, such as acculturation and language, are discussed, the more complex and less researched effects of systemic ethnocentrism and racism are also explored through multidisciplinary readings and discussions of the historical challenges related to citizenship and immigration, the context of racialization and the "forever foreigner" construction, and the place of

Asian American women in the dominant Black/White race dialogue within the United States (e.g., see Tuan, 1998).

Although information about and understanding of Asian American women is important, without addressing the second challenge of self-awareness, trainees may pathologize Asian American women clients because of their lack of awareness of the impact of their own worldviews and unconscious and unintended ethnocentrism, racism, or sexism. Non-Asian students of color and White European American students frequently share the first challenge, but their experiences of the second challenge are frequently different. For example, White European American students frequently enter CMH with limited awareness of how their own race and culture have affected their worldviews. They may adopt the view that because everyone's culture is different, everyone shares a similar status and copes with the same general issues. This view is frequently accompanied by the belief that because each client is different, the best way to approach being culturally sensitive is simply to learn from the client. In contrast, African American students frequently have significant awareness of how their own experiences of race and culture have affected their general worldviews and their interactions with White European Americans. However, they may still lack awareness about these issues in relation to interactions with Asian American women. They may see racialization as the primary influence on experience and conceptualize it as a Black-White dynamic, seeing Asian American women as much like White European Americans. They may be relatively unaware of the impacts of ethnicity and ethnocentrism (in addition to race and racism) on Asian American women.

Developing Self-Awareness: The Cultural Immersion Project

Finding ways to link the two goals of developing self-awareness *and* learning about others (e.g., Asian American women) in order to demonstrate their interdependence is a challenge for training. In CMH, the Cultural Immersion Project helps to address this challenge. Each student chooses one racial group or community upon which to focus, and may choose a particular subgroup within that racial group (e.g., a specific ethnicity such as Vietnamese, or another subgroup, such as Asian American women or Asian American gay men and lesbians). Students work collaboratively (i.e., at least two students focus on a particular cultural group together). The project consists of four "data collection" activities: (1) reading and critiquing the psychological research literature on the group; (2) interviewing individuals belonging to the group; (3) attending an event or community activity made up predominantly of members from the group; and (4) doing a "day in the life" exercise, imagining oneself as a member of the group and reflecting on how one's daily experience would be similar or different from one's usual experience. Each data collection activity is reflected upon in a journal, addressing not only what was experienced and what was learned about the people within the group, but also what was learned about one's own worldview, experiences, preconceptions, and biases. At the end of the project, students present what they have learned to the class and write a multi-part reflection paper, focusing on their own developing self-awareness.

The Cultural Immersion Project enables students to learn about others while positioning themselves in relation to those others (e.g., by reflecting on how they thought and felt while interviewing someone or attending a community event). It aims to address both the modal experience and the individual lived experience of Asian American women through exposure to both. It encourages students to consider social boundaries and critique socially constructed and agreed upon meanings by giving them multiple experiences with alternative social meanings from different sources. It requires that students focus upon the effects of their own experiences of oppression and privilege. It also enables students to experience a process of learning that can be utilized repeatedly throughout their training and career.

Developing Self-Awareness in Relation to Asian American Women: A Trainee's Perspective

> *The Cultural Immersion Project required that we make a "community visit" and write a journal entry about our experience. My initial reaction to this assignment was that it would be more challenging for me if: (1) I were European-American and; (2) I had not spent so much time with Asian Americans as friends, former roommates, dating partners, and social acquaintances. As an African American, I was confident that Asian Americans I encountered would, at least to a degree, perceive me as a fellow person of color, trust me, initiate interactions with me (or at a minimum, welcome me after I initiated an interaction), and feel some sense of alliance with me.*
>
> *My experience entering a neighborhood park filled with more than 80 Cambodian Americans (mostly males) and one African Ameri-*

can–me–could not have been further from my expectations. The individuals I approached would not maintain eye contact with me, gave terse answers to my questions, and quickly turned away from me. They adopted a posture that suggested mistrust, indifference, or subtle hostility. After several hours, when the first person to have a conversation with me that lasted longer than ten seconds was a young, acculturated, university-educated, Cambodian-ethnic woman, I felt apprehensive about how onlookers would evaluate my interaction with her and recognized an emerging consciousness about what a gendered space the park actually was.

What I took away from this experience combined with my other "data collection" activities and reflections was a heightened awareness that my cultural background, socioeconomic class, gender, sexual orientation, and beliefs are neither passive nor benign. Although I had not held a number of the dominant, mainstream stereotypic views about Asian American women, the lens through which I viewed them had been shaped by my own experiences, biases, and areas of privilege (i.e., being male, middle-class, and a U.S. citizen). Moreover, I realized that my presumptions about how I would be perceived by Asian American women and how I perceived them were based on interactions with acculturated females who were with me in mainstream spaces, and were not a representative sample of Asian-ethnic women.

When I met with my first Asian American female client, I remembered the crucial lessons I took away from CMH: (1) I did not assume that my client would immediately feel comfortable or allied with me or that I could accurately predict how she would perceive me. This stance is particularly important in my work with female clients for whom my status as a male, and the relative power and privilege associated with that status, might pose a threat and act as an obstacle to building a therapeutic alliance; (2) I remembered that there are substantial cultural differences among women self-identifying as Asian American, and that it would be irresponsible to assume homogeneity of values, beliefs, or perceptions across all peoples of Asian descent; and (3) I reminded myself that cultural sensitivity requires a continual commitment of time and energy and a willingness to be in spaces that do not feel comfortable.

APPLYING CULTURAL SENSITIVITY AND SELF-AWARENESS: INTERVENTION STRATEGIES

In the fall of their second year, students take Intervention Strategies (IS), a foundational course in psychotherapy theory and interventions, while also beginning their first supervised clinical practicum. An organizing assumption of the course is that effective therapy requires understanding the particular contexts, cultural traditions, and norms that have guided a client's development and are influencing her current functioning. The course aims to continue students' developmental journeys toward providing culturally sensitive therapy by: (1) integrating students' understandings of their own and others' cultural and systemic experiences with exposure to different therapeutic frameworks and their associated theories of personality and psychopathology (e.g., interpersonal psychodynamic, cognitive behavioral, emotion-focused); (2) continuing the development of students' reflexivity by explicitly examining the impact of their own backgrounds and positions on the process of establishing alliances with clients and on the relational dynamics of psychotherapy; and (3) providing structure and guidance for students beginning to apply culturally sensitive clinical skills in their first clinical practicum.

Understanding and Treating Asian American Women

The major challenges for trainees who are not Asian American in understanding and treating Asian American women at this point in their training are their circumscribed understanding of principles of therapy and ways of conceptualizing client problems, and their limited exposure to Asian American women clients. These issues together contribute to the potential to: (1) pay insufficient attention to the interaction of cultural context and theoretical conceptualization (and potentially to pathologize clients by misapplying Eurocentric frameworks in working with them); and/or (2) stereotype or overgeneralize from one Asian American female client to others and not be sufficiently appreciative of the full range of diversity among Asian American women. Students read additional theoretical information about Asian American women clients while class discussions and assignments focus on linking trainees' developing theoretical understandings and cultural sensitivity with actual clinical practice.

Building on the work done in CMH, in IS students learn to focus their attention on the multiple identities that characterize clients' and their own lives (e.g., being Asian American, female, working class, having a disability), the relative positions of privilege associated with those identities, the variable salience of those identities in different contexts, and the links between those identities and the ways in which clients conceptualize the problems that bring them into therapy. To reinforce this perspective, students read *Addressing Cultural Complexities in Clinical Practice* (Hays, 2001), a book that adopts a position on the combined importance of enhanced cultural self-understanding and understanding of diverse others similar to our own.

Integrating Theory, Practice, and Cultural Sensitivity

Two comparative intake assessment assignments encourage students to examine how theoretical frameworks and their own experiences affect their conceptualizations and treatment of clients. In the first assignment, trainees compare different theoretical frameworks. Trainees write up two initial intake assessments of the same client they are currently seeing employing: (1) the Addressing Framework focusing on the client's multiple cultural identities articulated by Hays (2001); and (2) the Interpersonal Psychodynamic Framework articulated by Luborsky (Book, 1998). Trainees reflect on the ways in which each framework contributes to their understanding of the client, the information attended to and ignored when working with the client, the treatment plan adopted, and their emerging alliance with the client. In the second assignment, trainees write and compare two additional intake summaries, one on a client that they perceive to be similar to them culturally and one on a client they perceive to be quite different. They then reflect on the experience of doing these two assessments and their process of initiating psychotherapy with these two clients, including the depth of their understanding of the clients and the ease with which they are engaging the clients in treatment. A trainee may reflect, for example, on her ability to form a therapeutic alliance with a client who, like her, is a woman, but who is an Asian American who grew up in a different country, speaks English as a second language, and is significantly older than she. This assignment invites students to think critically about who they are and how their multiple identities shape the relationship that is unfolding between them and their clients. It also encourages them to consider how their clients view themselves in the world, how they may expect to be treated by others who are different from them, and how they may behave in unfamiliar situations such as an initial therapy session with a therapist with particular social identities. Finally, it helps student therapists identify areas where their knowledge is incomplete. Trainees are expected to assume responsibility for educating themselves about the larger historical and cultural meanings of a client's multiple identities (e.g., the history and politics associated with being a 50-year-old female Vietnamese refugee).

Limited exposure to clients generally (e.g., students carry a caseload of only 4-5 clients in their first practicum) and to Asian American female clients in particular presents challenges because our aim is for all students to be able to provide culturally sensitive therapy to Asian American women. Discussions of published case materials (e.g., case studies in Chin, Liem, Hong, & Ham, 1993) and case presentations by students working with Asian American female clients are particularly important in addressing this challenge. To emphasize heterogeneity and the importance of avoiding overgeneralization, discussions focus explicitly on how a given case example is both similar to the group modal experience and particular to this individual, as well as on issues related to applying a given theoretical model and treatment strategy to Asian American women clients similar to and different from the particular case examples. To emphasize reflexivity, students are invited to imagine themselves as the therapist and to consider how their own gender, race, and culture might interact with those of the particular client. Through these case discussions, even students who are not currently seeing an Asian American woman client may reflect on how they might work effectively with that particular individual. An example of the work done by one student therapist with one Asian woman follows.

INTEGRATING THEORY, PRACTICE, AND CULTURAL SENSITIVITY WITH ASIAN AMERICAN WOMEN: A TRAINEE'S PERSPECTIVE

I am a 24-year-old, third-generation-Italian-American, monolingual (English only) female therapist. Eungie was a 29-year-old female Korean international student who spoke English as a second language. She sought therapy because of anxiety and depression associated with what she conceived of as a physical disability–she experienced muscle stiffness that made her academic work difficult.

With Eungie, I used the ADDRESSING Framework to explore the personal meanings of Eungie's multiple roles and identities, and her understanding of her difficulties and the process of therapy. In Eungie's case, it was particularly important to consider the intersections of race, gender, culture, and ability/disability and the multiple related life adjustments she was experiencing in returning to school and coming to the U.S. Eungie felt isolated from her peers and other potential support systems because of her nationality, language, culture, race, age and a disability that had become compounded by the fact that her courses were now in English.

My first session with Eungie was very anxiety provoking for me. I had to consciously think about the rate of my speech and the words I was using–something I had never done before. At times I would ask a question and Eungie would silently tilt her head to the side in a questioning manner. Her eyes seemed to say, "I want to answer you but I don't know what you mean." When she did answer, many doubts ran through my mind–Did she understand the question? Did I understand her answer? Were we really talking about the same thing? I was aware that the barrier between us was not imposed by Eungie's lack of knowing any English, but by my lack of knowing any Korean. She knew both of our languages, and I only knew mine. I was conscious of the need to build an alliance, a sense that we were working together. I decided to verbalize the difficulty we were having communicating and suggested that sometimes it might take us a few tries to help one another understand what we were trying to say. At the end of our first session, I asked her what it had been like for her to talk to a White therapist who conducted the sessions in English. Eungie thought for a moment and said, "Sometimes it was hard, but it will be okay." I told her I would be happy to continue working with her, but I would also be happy to help her find a therapist who could speak Korean if that made more sense to her. To my surprise, she said, "I would like to stay here and talk to you."

During our work together, I was conscious of the fact that Eungie and I initially had different views about the purpose of psychotherapy and the nature of her difficulties. Eungie's experience was that she was struggling with a physical disability that caused her stress and anxiety and affected her academic performance (rather than an anxiety disorder causing physical difficulties). Furthermore, Eungie did not consider it appropriate to talk at length about her emotions in therapy, nor did she feel she could fully express these emotions in English. I knew that engaging Eungie in therapy would be facilitated if I respected her understanding of what was going on and her preferences for treatment. I therefore focused on making sure she got the services and support she needed at school (tutoring, extra time on tests, etc.) and on teaching relaxation techniques to help manage her anxiety. Our comfort with one another and with the nature of our work together grew and, in time, Eungie's anxiety lessened and her academic performance improved considerably giving her a sense of empowerment and confidence.

INTEGRATING CULTURAL SENSITIVITY WITH COMMUNITY PRACTICE

Most students complete their second clinical practicum in community hospitals or health/mental health centers that are committed to serving culturally diverse and underserved populations. Several sites in the greater Boston area serve a significant number of Asian American clients, including a site in Boston's Chinatown that serves primarily urban Asian and Southeast Asian immigrant clients. As is the case for other racial/ethnic groups, it is usually Asian women (rather than men) who seek out services either for themselves or for their children.

Understanding and Treating Asian American Women

Major challenges for trainees treating Asian American women at this stage of their training include integrating and applying culturally sensitive understandings, processes, and skills they have learned while working within systems that may not always emphasize a cultural perspective. The development of a critical, comparative, systemic approach to their training and practice within a changing health-care system is emphasized in the yearlong seminar associated with the community practicum. Students working with Asian American women are challenged to think about the systems of care available to these women and the goodness of fit between clients' needs and ways of conceptualizing their problems, and the services available to them and how those services are organized.

Clinical experiences encountered in the community reveal how important the developmental process outlined in this article is in developing cultural sensitivity. This is illustrated in the following example offered by a White European American student about her community practicum experience.

Working Within Community Systems to Treat Asian American Women: A Trainee's Perspective

I worked with Xiang, a 32-year-old Chinese American mother, at an outpatient community mental health center that serves mostly ethnic minority clients who are economically disadvantaged and frequently involved with multiple systems (e.g., Department of Social Services [DSS], schools, other therapists, physicians, homeless shelters). Xiang, her husband, and her three children (7, 9, and 10) were referred from DSS after several domestic violence incidents had been reported by neighbors. Xiang's husband became violent when disagreements arose. Xiang hit her children when they disrespected her and repeatedly yelled at them that they would be "failures" or "losers" when they did not obey her. Two days before I met Xiang, the court had ordered her to leave the family home and live elsewhere.

In a strong Chinese accent, Xiang's first words to me were "I hope you help, because everyone against me, even my family." She kept her coat on despite the warm temperature in the room and told me in a pressured and angry stream of words about her current homeless situation as she fingered her large duffel bag that she had placed on her lap between us. As I listened to her, I realized I was surprised that she did not fit the "submissive" Asian woman stereotype and then I felt angry at myself that this thought had entered my head. I realized that my emotions and thoughts were linked to my desire to help and my gnawing fear of incompetence that was part of my internal consciousness especially when I began to work with a new client of different racial, cultural or class background than me. Because Xiang expressed many convictions about parenting, I asked her about her life when she was growing up. I could not have predicted that she had spent her teenage years in Africa and that she had invested all her energy in her studies to please her parents and avoid feeling like an outsider based on her ethnicity and race. Hearing about her unique experience of coming of age in Africa as an Asian woman with strict parents helped me to consider how her values and worldview starkly contrasted with those of her children who were being raised in the U.S. Adopting a respectful curiosity about her experiences appeared to facilitate her own reflections about the manner in which she was parented and the ways in which she was currently trying to discipline her children.

By the time I met Xiang, she had experienced extensive anxiety and depression for some time. In addition, she had encountered prejudice when involved with systems of care and was mistrustful of people in the "helping professions" who were in positions of authority. She spoke openly about DSS workers having a "conspiracy" against her and about how her husband gambled away his salary despite her objections. To work effectively with Xiang, I relied on my learning and understanding that females may have less power within traditional Asian families, particularly those that are economically disadvantaged, and may be expected to fulfill specific gender roles such as tending the house and raising the children. I knew that immigrant parents may face additional challenges such as a limited social support network of people who share their bicultural experience of raising children in the U.S. who tend to adopt American values more readily than the values of their parents. My training facilitated my conceptualization of Xiang's behavior and emotions via the lens of power.

At a meeting with other mental health workers involved in working with the family, DSS personnel and Xiang's housing advocate, Xiang was described by one person as "bordering on psychotic." Xiang's use of trigger words such as "conspiracy" and repeated use of "they" without a specific reference group contributed to this interpretation. One person who was extremely frustrated with her refusal to leave the family home (so that her children could live there with her husband) suggested severely reducing the frequency of her supervised visitation until she complied with these demands. Without consideration of context, her behavior seemed irrational. Given her past experience in which cooperation with her violent husband meant acceptance of her lack of power and her discriminatory experiences with service providers, however, her behavior appeared strategic and adaptive. She could not afford housing for herself and she did not trust her husband to appropriately parent her children. Discussing her behavior and substantial anxiety in the context of past trauma helped the group adopt a more empathic attitude towards her and consider ways to facilitate cooperation with Xiang and supervised visitation for Xiang and her children.

THE ONGOING NATURE OF BECOMING CULTURALLY SENSITIVE

Training therapists to work effectively with Asian American women clients involves fostering in them a heightened awareness of how their multiple social systemic identities and statuses–their race, culture, gender, social class, age, etc.–have affected their worldviews, their approaches to and expectations about relationships, and their values and judgments about health and pathology. Understanding biases and assumptions rooted in the dominant discourse that one may not initially be aware of, but which have nonetheless been internalized, is especially key, as demonstrated by the interactions described previously between an African American male graduate student and male and female Cambodian immigrants. The race discourse in the U.S. emphasizes White (on one "side") and "people of color" (on the other). From his own lived experiences and his experiences with this discourse, this African American student expected all Asian Americans to see him as "like them" and was surprised when the Cambodian refugees in the park saw him as "other." Experiencing and reflecting upon his own assumptions through the cultural immersion project helped him avoid imposing them on his female client and developed in him an essential sensitivity to the heterogeneity of Asian American women.

Successful treatment of Asian American women involves the integration of self-awareness, cultural knowledge about these women (and their within-group differences), and theoretical frameworks into culturally sensitive case conceptualizations and treatment plans. The training in CMH and IS helped Eungie's therapist think critically about different theoretical frameworks and their applicability in Eungie's case. It also helped her incorporate Eungie's own culturally-related conceptualizations of her difficulties, that were initially different than the therapist's, into the conceptualization of the presenting problem and the approach to treating it. Similarly, Xiang's therapist's training experiences gave her practice in seeing the influence of gender, culture, race, and power on her client's developing difficulties. Her understanding of how social systemic variables affect Asian American women clients was crucial to her problem conceptualization and treatment strategy.

Successful treatment with Asian American women also requires linking culturally sensitive conceptualizations with skills and interventions that also reflect self-awareness and knowledge of Asian American women. Forming cross-cultural alliances involves anticipating possible cultural or other systemic disconnections in the therapy process (e.g., due to language, race, gender differences) and feeling comfortable addressing these disconnections in a way that creates alliance, not defensiveness. Self-awareness of and comfort with their own racial, cultural, and/or language privilege enabled all three training therapists to address these issues directly. Their direct communications about differences between themselves and their clients increased the confidence felt by their Asian American women clients that they were being respected and understood by their therapists and contributed to their active engagement in treatment. Xiang's therapist's training not only affected her thinking and conceptualization, but also gave her needed practice in articulating this understanding, enabling her to intervene at the systemic level with other service providers. Framing what others saw as Xiang's paranoia and stubbornness as a response to repeated experiences of powerlessness (connected to gender, culture, and race) not only contributed to the individual therapist's alliance with Xiang, but also enabled other providers to empathize more and consider alternative meanings and interventions.

Training students to provide culturally sensitive care to Asian American women means nurturing within them a commitment to ongoing learning. Developing cultural understanding, heightened self-awareness, and culturally appropriate clinical skills is a lifelong process; the case examples provided previously by the three trainees illustrate how training experiences build upon one another. Coursework that encourages self-awareness; focuses on understanding the impact of culture on values, relationships, and behaviors; and explicitly attends to the influence of structural inequities related to race and gender, motivates students to embrace the process of continually expanding their self-awareness, acquiring new knowledge, and recognizing the current limits of their understanding. Ongoing engagement with this cyclical process is further fueled by trainees' recognition that cultural sensitivity is a prerequisite for ethical and efficacious treatment with Asian American women. Successful training assists students in seeing clearly the clinical need for and essential benefits of culturally sensitive practice.

REFERENCES

American Psychological Association (2003). Guidelines on multicultural education, training, research, practice, and organizational change for psychologists. *American Psychologist, 58*, 377-402.

Arredondo, P., Toporek, R., Brown, S. P., Jones, J., Locke, D. C., Sanchez, J., & Stadler, H. (1996). Operationalization of the multicultural counseling competencies. *Journal of Multicultural Counseling and Development, 24*, 42-78.

Atkinson, D. R., Morten, G., & Sue, D. W. (Eds.) (1998). *Counseling American minorities.* Boston: McGraw Hill.

Book, Howard (1998). *How to practice brief psychodynamic psychotherapy: The core conflictual relationship theme method.* Washington, DC: American Psychological Association.

Chin, J. L. (Ed.) (2000). *Relationships among Asian American women.* Washington, DC: American Psychological Association.

Chin, J., Liem, J., Ham, M., & Hong, G. (Eds.) (1993). *Transference and empathy in Asian American psychotherapy: Culture, values, and treatment needs.* Westport, CT: Praeger.

Chung, R. H. G. (2001). Gender, ethnicity, and acculturation in intergenerational conflict of Asian American college students. *Cultural Diversity and Mental Health, 7,* 376-386.

Cox, S. S. (Ed.) (1999). *Voices from another place: A collection of works from a generation born in Korea and adopted to other countries.* St. Paul, MN: Yeong & Yeong Book Company.

Eng, P. (1995). Domestic violence in Asian/Pacific Island communities: A public health issue. In D. L. Adams (Ed.), *Health issues for women of color: A cultural diversity perspective.* Thousand Oaks, CA: Sage.

Hays, P. (2001). *Addressing cultural complexities in practice.* Washington, DC: American Psychological Association.

Lee, J. F. J. (1992). *Asian Americans: Oral histories of first to fourth generation Americans from China, the Philippines, Japan, India, the Pacific Islands, Vietnam and Cambodia*, New York: New Press.

Root, M. P. P. (1995). The psychology of Asian American women. In H. Landrine (Ed.), *Bringing cultural diversity to feminist psychology: Theory, research, and practice.* Washington, DC: American Psychological Association.

Root, M. P. P. (1998). Women. In L. C. Lee & N. W. S. Zane (Eds.), *Handbook of Asian American psychology* (pp. 211-231). Thousand Oaks, CA: Sage.

Sue, D. W., & Sue, D. (2002). *Counseling the culturally diverse: Theory and practice* (4th ed.). New York: Wiley.

Thai, H. C. (2002). Clashing dreams: Highly educated overseas brides and low-wage U.S. husbands. In B. Ehrenreich & A. R. Hochschild (Eds.), *Global women.* New York: Metropolitan Books.

Tuan, M. (1998). *Forever foreigners or honorary Whites.* New Brunswick, NJ: Rutgers University Press.

U.S. Department of Health and Human Services (2001). *Mental health: Culture, race, and ethnicity–A supplement to mental health: A report of the Surgeon General.* Rockville, MD: U.S. Department of Health and Human Services, Public Health Service, Office of the Surgeon General.

Uba, L. (1994). *Asian Americans: Personality patterns, identity, and mental health.* New York: Guilford Press.

Weber, L. (2000). *Understanding race, class, gender and sexuality: A conceptual framework.* New York: McGraw-Hill.

doi:10.1300/J015v30n03_15

Index

For Product Safety Concerns and Information please contact our EU representative GPSR@taylorandfrancis.com
Taylor & Francis Verlag GmbH, Kaufingerstraße 24, 80331 München, Germany

www.ingramcontent.com/pod-product-compliance
Lightning Source LLC
LaVergne TN
LVHW011125300926
849160LV00008B/511
9780789034342